WHEN THE GIRLS CAME OUT TO PLAY

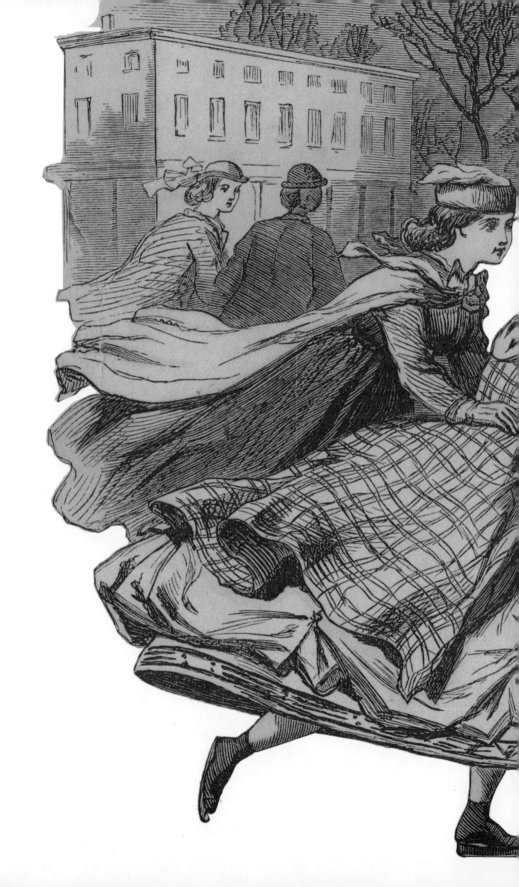

WHEN THE GIRLS CAME OUT TO PLAY

The Birth of American Sportswear

Patricia Campbell Warner

UNIVERSITY OF MASSACHUSETTS PRESS
Amherst and Boston

LC 2006003037
ISBN 1-55849-548-7 (library cloth ed.); 549-5 (paper)

Designed by Sally Nichols
Set in Monotype Walbaum
Printed and bound by The Maple-Vail Manufacturing Group

Library of Congress Cataloging-in-Publication Data

Warner, Patricia Campbell, 1936–
    When the girls came out to play : the birth of American sportswear / Patricia
Campbell Warner.
        p. cm.
    Includes bibliographical references and index.
    ISBN 1-55849-549-5 (pbk. : alk. paper)—ISBN 1-55849-548-7 (library cloth :
alk. paper)
    1. Sport clothes for women—United States—History—20th century.   2. Sports
for women—United States—History—20th century.   I. Title.
    GT1855.W37 2006
    391'.209730904—dc22

                                                                                  2006003037

British Library Cataloguing in Publication data are available.

CONTENTS

CONTENTS

ILLUSTRATIONS

ILLUSTRATIONS

ILLUSTRATIONS

PREFACE

OVER THE YEARS AS I WORKED ON THE TOPIC OF WOMEN, SPORTS, AND THE clothing devised for exercise in the nineteenth and early twentieth centuries, people would ask me how I got interested in the topic. They usually assumed that I was athletic myself, and the interest sprang from that. Those who knew me well knew this was not the case. The only reason I had participated in sports or athletics in high school was—typical of teenagers everywhere—because my friends did. These were the mid-twentieth-century years, when girls wore their baggy romper-leg cotton gym suits to play basketball and volleyball, and, if they were lucky, got to wear shorts to play games such as badminton. Generally speaking, sports for girls were disregarded, though my school was better than most. We had no outdoor field, no track, no pool, but we were fortunate to have our own Girls' Gym, separated from the Boys' Gym by wide doors that scarcely kept out the deep shouts that emanated from the boys' side. And we did have two women gym teachers who created what they called a "Leaders' Group" to encourage girls to play non-curricular games such as archery and badminton and to learn how to referee basketball and volleyball in the loose athletic league of nearby schools. Only much, much later in my life did I understand how unusual this was in that era. This was not a period when girls were encouraged to love playing sports.

So how did I end up devoting years of my life to this study? The answer is simple. However unwittingly, a friend got me into it. Indeed, it could justifiably be claimed that I followed the same passive pattern established early in my life—certainly by high school. When I was a graduate student studying design at the University of Minnesota, a fellow student, Otto Thieme, recommended me to the university art museum as a possible speaker to accompany a traveling exhibition being planned. Apparently the organizers thought that a talk centered on clothing would give a different twist, and at the time I was the student who was studying the history of dress. The exhibition was to go out a year or more hence and would travel for two years. I would fly to each of the towns on the schedule to give my talk. Since I was working three-quarter time, doing the course work for my Ph.D., was the mother of two teenage sons, and was going through a divorce, this sounded like a pleasant distraction. Not committing myself, I went to look at the prints being readied for the show. They ranged in period from 1860 to 1940 and dealt with the broad theme of leisure, of American pastimes. It was titled "America at Play."

As I looked at the prints the staff had chosen, I realized that unless I could narrow the focus (the Design Department taught us to identify variables, establish limitations, and work within them), I would be discussing the entire range of clothing for both men and women in that eighty-year period—not a good thing. I offered instead to talk about the clothing for sports. Great! they said. Whatever you like! So, pleased with myself and happy that I had a year or more to work on this, I hied myself to the university library to find all the books I could on sports clothing, and women's clothing for sports in particular. Of course, I expected a subsection devoted to the subject within the general clothing and fashion holdings, and assumed that the next year or so would be a merry round of reading light and interesting books on the subject. Instead, I found nothing. A few brief mentions peppered general histories of dress; usually they were arch and jocular, and were illustrated with a picture or two of women wearing impossible clothing—hats, hoops, bustles, corsets, long skirts—to play croquet or tennis, or to go bathing. Apart from that, nothing. The approaching months took on an entirely different aspect.

I could have gone back to the idea of a general survey of dress during the eighty years in question, but that idea left me unmoved. It became a challenge, a game almost, to find sources. My memories of that time are of sitting on the cold cement floor in the bowels of the University of Minnesota

Comstock Library, pulling out nineteenth-century magazines whose edges gently crumbled in my hands and onto my clothing as I gingerly opened and read them, searching for any references to participation in outdoor games and sports. I would lose myself in them, emerging hours later with the gems I had collected that day, tired but happy. Eventually I assembled enough for my traveling talk, which I illustrated with a collection of slides I had made.

I ventured forth in little aircraft on often bumpy flights to towns and small cities in the Upper Midwest to talk to local art groups about what women in the past had worn when they wanted to participate in vigorous sport or exercise. I was astounded at the response. After listening politely, women wanted to share their own memories, and invariably began reminiscing about the gym suits they had worn. They would end up talking to one another, more or less ignoring me, sparking memories and laughter as they animatedly described their outfits and their activities. In some of the audiences elderly ladies regaled us with tales of baggy black bloomers and stockings, middy blouses, and big hair ribbons ("Oh, look, Mabel! Do you remember that? That picture is just like what I wore!"). Others recalled the blue rompers, the green camp shorts and shirts of a later period. All this reminiscing came pouring out in spite of the fact that I had little more than mentioned the whole phenomenon of gym wear and related activities in my talk. To my mind, that was an entirely different category of clothing from what I was there to discuss—clothing for sport. But listening to those women, I was struck by the common experience, the common memory, the laughter and nostalgia that invariably accompanied their personal stories.

It took, all told, over three years before I finished my involvement with the art museum. From this vantage point, I realize that those years, perhaps more than any other aspect of my graduate education, taught me creative research techniques and gave me invaluable public speaking experience. They also gave me, through the reminiscences of my audiences, insight into a facet of my work that I might otherwise have taken far longer to come to. I loved doing it and was sorry when it was over. For one thing, it spelled the end of my excuse for not completing my degree.

Towards the end of the period when I was actively lecturing for the art museum, my adviser, Timothy Blade, a decorative arts specialist who had left me on my own for years, finally paid me a visit to find out how my dissertation was coming along. I had to confess that it wasn't. At all. I had had a perfect topic picked out for years, but kept bumping into all sorts of problems with it. He looked at me in exasperation, then demanded, "Well, what about all this sports stuff you've been doing for the past two years? That's all original research, isn't it? Why don't you just use that?" I remember gaping at him, thunderstruck, and thinking this "sports stuff" was way too much fun to turn into a dissertation. But within about a minute after he left my office, I knew he was right. I knew that I had found my topic. Or, rather, he had identified it for me. So here, finally, officially, and very belatedly, especially since both, alas, are dead, I acknowledge the indelible influence those two men, Otto Thieme and Tim Blade, had on my life.

I mention this story because we all too often ignore passing opportunities that can, if we act on them, literally change our lives. I sense that none of the intervening years would have played out as they did had I dismissed Otto and Tim and their suggestions. As it was, I wrote the dissertation, got my degree, and moved on into academia. In the process, I came to understand one of the greatest truisms of all, that we are happiest in our work if we choose to do the things that don't feel like work to us, the things that we spend our spare time thinking about.

In a perfect world, I would have written the book based on my dissertation years ago, as I had fully intended to. But in retrospect I must confess I'm glad that circumstances prevented me from doing it earlier. I am grateful to have had twenty years to let the subject roil, settle, re-form, and eventually grow to make new connections in my head. It simply takes time for me to let myself think. And I have found that, even though I have wanted to leave the topic alone over the years, it would not let me be. It has kept nudging me with new information, with new links and ideas. Only very recently have I felt it was time to sit down and write what I know about women, sports and exercise, and clothing.

The other influence on my thinking about clothing for sport and exercise goes much deeper in my consciousness and my past. It stems from my lifelong interest in the clothing of ordinary people—people like me. As a girl growing up, I loved clothes. My mother often told me that her mother, my grandmother, was aghast and dismayed that she let me choose my own clothes from a very early age. Apparently even as a little girl I had strong likes and dislikes, and a strong sense of how I should dress. (Today, in an era of TV, magazines, malls, and the ferocious sales pitch, that behavior seems to be more common among children than not, but in the 1940s and early 1950s it was unusual. Mothers, I think, had greater control then.) As I grew older, I loved thinking about clothes, planning them, shopping for patterns and fabric, and making them. I particularly loved imagining outfits in my mind's eye, then putting the pieces together to create them. I loved wearing combinations that nobody else had. Early on, my parents had put me on an allowance, which eventually, from about the time I was twelve, became a clothes allowance. This was one of the reasons why I learned to sew. Not only did I have a body that no ready-made clothing fit properly (who doesn't?), but I soon realized that I could have a lot more to wear if I was willing to make my clothes myself. I saved up and learned to be canny with my money. It's a habit that has lasted throughout my life. Of course, the other part—the part that says if you can get great clothes cheap, you can have a lot more of them—has kept my closets clogged for years.

I think I was in high school when I became aware of the "Best Dressed" lists. Each year, women's fashion magazines would choose the Best Dressed. They were—are—invariably rich, glossy women, groomed within an inch of their lives (especially in the 1950s). They wore designer clothes in the days when that meant something, the true haute couture. I clearly remember wondering why those women deserved the title. It seemed to me that they had found a designer who could fit them well (they all looked slim and beautiful—easy to fit), but they went with *his* look rather than their own. *They* didn't have to do a thing but go to a couturier and passively be dressed by him, in his style. Of course, this is still true, as any copy of *Vogue* will attest. So-and-so in an Oscar de la Renta, Somebody in a Ralph or a Calvin. For the life of me, I couldn't understand why, just because they were rich, these women deserved the credit and the adulation. Theirs were not the taste, the selection, the planning, the work: theirs was the money. And after all, the designers were just doing their job, giving Mrs. One-Percent-of-the-Population her suave, sophisticated elegance. In effect, she played Galatea to the designer's Pygmalion. No, it seemed to me that the women who really deserved credit were the average, ordinary women who, like me, managed on a small budget to put together wonderful, flattering outfits that cost next to nothing. One could see them every day on the city streets—smart, attractive, eye-catching women who had a knack for clothes and great personal style. Surely they were the ones deserving a Best

Dressed label. And surely I wasn't the only girl who had such thoughts. I was convinced that the Best Dressed *really were* people like me. Creative. Thrifty. In love with clothes.

As I grew older and wiser, I realized that there was more to it than that. Nevertheless, the more democratic interest in clothing the masses rather than the elite few stuck. It lasted well into middle age, during the period I was becoming a costume historian. And it is still with me. No surprise, then, that the focus of my work has always been on the clothing of ordinary people. Many writers concentrate on the designers or on the novel in dress; they write beautifully illustrated books on all aspects of high fashion. I am grateful to them because they have informed me and my teaching. But I have always been more interested in how our clothes got to be the way they are. I am interested in the struggle women have had to wear clothing that made sense. I wanted to find out where that clothing came from, what the precursors were to the comfortable clothing that the world knows today as American sportswear. This book tells that story.

When I finished writing my dissertation some twenty years ago, the study of clothing in the United States was generally held in relatively low regard by the academic community. Only now has this begun to change. A new, vital study of dress is extending beyond the traditional clothing and textiles programs of what used to be called home economics and moving into departments such as history, art history, and even economics. Scholars are beginning to look at clothing and its social implications in new ways. Costume exhibitions in major museums have had strong influence on the acceptance of costume studies; indeed, the most popular exhibitions, the ones that bring in the largest audiences, are quite often those, like the internationally successful Jacqueline Kennedy exhibition, that display clothes. Nothing, it would seem, is more evocative of time and place or can reach an audience more directly than clothing. It is something we all have in common, and we share a common memory of styles, looks, personalities. Museums have helped create an atmosphere of interest and enthusiasm for the study.

The British have been the leaders in the field of costume history since its beginning. Indeed, until recently, most of the major writers have been British, so most of the points of view in the field are also British. As a result, when Americans have written about clothing, they have incorporated into their work the English antecedents and English tone, even English examples, which may or may not reflect America and its culture. There is even a tendency to interchange one for the other. In my opinion this is a mistake, since both the histories and the clothing are very different. As Americans, we developed our own "look" in clothing, however closely it parallels a more universal fashion. Today, though, more than ever before in history, because of instant international communication through movies, television, and the Web, people everywhere are closer to becoming one huge, unified, dressed-alike mass. There are outlets of the same clothing stores in Europe and America, even in Asia. And yet the differences still linger. They may be subtle, more so all the time, as in the quality of fabrics, or the cut and attention to the body underneath, the angles of the seams or the height of the crotch, or even the way of putting clothes together. But the differences are there. Because I grew up in Canada, in close contact with the United States, these differences between people who are "the same" have always intrigued me. Today it is virtually impossible to tell Canadians and Americans apart from the clothes they wear. But because of all these factors, I am interested in American clothing—not British and American, or "Western dress," but the clothing that is expressive of American women, of American development, of American society. And no clothing is more expressive of American women than American sportswear.

Ultimately, certainly among many academics, the question arises, why bother studying clothing at all? It is almost invariably regarded as frivolous. Clothing can be a headache, a source of anxiety or self-consciousness, a cause of despair, a reason for envy, a focus of contention, a wrap of anonymity. Those of us who study it use those very reasons for justifying its consideration. In the last analysis, however, clothing is necessary. Everyone in the world uses it in some form or another. Yet if it were simply a necessity, it would not carry negative connotations. It would be accepted routinely, like tooth-brushing, and be forgotten. Instead, it is much more than that: a source of personal expression in a world that conspires increasingly to limit our individuality, a means of personal pleasure, joy, and pride. It tells others who we are, what we represent. It can hint at a mind no longer connecting cleanly, or one dominated by conservatism or delusions of grandeur, by whimsy or daring. It also represents billions of dollars a year in this country alone: women's apparel sales in 2000 reached $96.6 billion.

The clothing we wear today is the result of the accumulated clothing of our past. As society has evolved to its present state, so has clothing, borrowing from past centuries and periods, always changing, always expressing the contemporary—and always being interpreted through contemporary eyes and sensibilities. As it is in constant flux, it is an expression of fashion in whatever time, whatever place. That is the nature of fashion. But fashion is a process that affects all aspects of a changing society, not just dress but architecture, language, science, philosophy, economics, war. Fashion has become an object of scorn only because it has been almost exclusively associated with women's clothing. The common understanding seems to be that women wear fashions, fashions keep changing, therefore fashion demands a mindless, slavish following even in a period, like today, of "free choice." As with lunches, though, there is no free choice. To resist fashion is to move counter-culture, which in itself may be regarded as an expression of fashion, since in the counter-culture it is fashionable to be non-fashionable. Fashion turns all aspects of society even as society turns fashion.

Despite that—or, better, in conjunction with it—certain periods of history have reflected major change. In other words, within a relatively brief span of time, the fashion of a nation can turn from one expression to another one vastly different. The period I am interested in, mainly from the 1860s up to World War II, is one of those times. Indeed, it may represent the greatest change in the shortest time frame in the history of the world. It is well known that war acts as a natural agent of change. But other factors too are involved in the process—or, rather, the factors leading to war may well influence other areas that are less well observed, and effect sweeping changes in places far removed from the battlefields. It is here, then, away from the significant male-oriented events of the nineteenth and twentieth centuries, that this book belongs. My interest centers on the women of the period, who, like the men, were undergoing a process of great change during these years. And their clothing reflected that change throughout.

This was the period that saw the establishment and growth of women's higher education in the United States. The United States led the way for the world in its thrust to recognize the worth of women's education, a significant but little-recognized accomplishment. Coming out of a period when women were regarded as home- and family-bound, the vision and determination of a few resolute women such as Mary Lyon, Catharine Beecher, and Sarah Josepha Hale are truly remarkable. The Susan B. Anthonys and Elizabeth Cady Stantons are well recognized today, but the foundations of education for women were already under way by the time the women's suffrage movement was established in the late 1840s. Without that acceptance of the need to educate women, and the right of women to be educated, the support for women's rights might have been even slower than it was to gain a foothold in the society of the era.

The girls who were sent off to school to be educated like their brothers were being sent away from home, often for the first time. The women who ran the schools tried to incorporate all the activities they felt necessary to mold a fully rounded graduate. That included physical activity. But what clothing did a girl wear for this when she may never have been encouraged to do anything like it before? Indeed, what choices did she have? And how did the clothing that eventually emerged for exercise relate to the dress worn outside the educational environment, perhaps for playing one of the new games that became so popular at the same time? The links between sports, clothing, and women's higher education are profound, entwined to the point of fusion. There is no doubt that, by looking at women's lives through the medium of their clothing, we can trace the slow emergence from the close restrictiveness of the early Victorian age to the acceptance of women's participation in a broader society during the eighty years under review.

Interestingly, of the vast numbers of books on sport and its history, even in the rare ones that mention women, no serious mention is made of the clothing women wore to participate. Yet women's involvement in athletics, like men's, was shaped by the freedom of movement permitted by the clothes they wore. What was possible for them was constrained by the swathing of their fashionable dress and the equally hampering expectations of their place in society. And women embraced all these limitations wholeheartedly. It was usually women themselves who professed the greatest shock at behavior considered unsuitable for a lady. Men had simplified their dress for sports early on beginning in the mid-nineteenth century, when they softened their shirt collars, donned the new rubber-soled shoes, shucked off their jackets, wore knickerbockers or other loose trousers, and played actively to their hearts' delight. They wore figure-revealing knit swimsuits and no one cared. By the end of the century they wore cotton trousers, had cut the legs off to make shorts, had cut out the sleeves to make what we now call tank tops, and ran bare-legged and barefoot in their light running shoes. They had done this by the time of the first modern Olympic Games in Athens in 1896, and they were hailed as gods. But the women? As we will see, they were permitted none of these things. They were not even considered as contestants in those first modern Games, and when they did show up for the second Olympics in Paris in 1900, they were included almost by mistake. There they wore their street clothes to play golf. It would take almost another century before women equalized the odds. And clothing has always played a significant part.

Little if anything has been written to throw light on the story of women and the clothing they devised for athletics and exercise. This book will attempt to fill that gap.

Several chapters in this book have been revised from articles published elsewhere, and I thank the editors and publishers for permission to use this material here. "The Gym Suit: Freedom at Last," in Patricia A. Cunningham, ed., *Dress in American Culture* (Madison: University of Wisconsin Press); "Clothing as Barrier: American Women in the Olympics, 1900–1920," *Dress* 24 (1977): 55–68, by permission of the Costume Society of America; "The Comely Rowers: The Beginnings of Collegiate Sports Uniforms for Women Crew at Wellesley, 1876–1900," *Clothing and Textiles Research Journal* 10, no. 3 (1992): 64–75, by permission of the International Textile & Apparel Association; Patricia Campbell Warner and Margaret S. Ewing, "Wading in the Water: Women Aquatic Biologists Coping with Clothing, 1877–1945," *BioScience* 52, no. 1 (January 2002), copyright, American Institute of Biological Sciences.

Over the years, I have visited many libraries and archives in the United States, Canada, England, and France and have received great help from them. Foremost among these are Mount Holyoke College Archives and Special Collections and the wonderful Patricia Albright, who has been there for as long as I have been doing this work. Thanks, too, go to Wilma Slaight at Wellesley College's Archives. Other collections important to my research were Smith and Vassar Colleges, the Universities of Michigan, California Berkeley, Toronto, and Minnesota. Many other collections provided information that eventually fleshed out the story I wanted to tell. I am a devoted fan of the talent and knowledge of the librarians and archivists at these institutions, quite apart from my admiration for the collections that they represent.

The College of Human Ecology at the University of Minnesota, the University of Massachusetts Amherst, and USDA Hatch Grants provided funds for my work over the years. Further thanks go to Harley Erdman, Lee Edwards, Paul Kostecki, and Cleve Willis of UMass Amherst. I am grateful for their support. In addition, I can't thank enough the staff at the University of Massachusetts Press, especially Clark Dougan, Carol Betsch, and Sally Nichols, and my copy editor, Amanda Heller, for their kindness, encouragement, and enthusiasm throughout the entire process of publishing this book.

With a work like this which has taken some twenty years of my life to birth, there are too many people to thank individually. Over the years, so many have sent along clippings of girls in gym suits, of early basketball teams, of girls wearing bloomers and black stockings, of Victorian women doing calisthenics and exercises. I hope they will allow me to thank them all in this very general way. I have appreciated their help more than I can say, and their interest in my work even more.

A special mention must be given to the Costume Society of America and the members who have encouraged me ever since I was a graduate student to share my findings. (Encouraged is hardly the word. More like "When are you ever going to write that book?") CSA has been a joy of my life, a prop to me in troubled times, and the source of some of my warmest friendships. More important, it has provided an outlet for my professional work, both at symposiums and in its journal, *Dress*. I particularly want to thank Trish Cunningham, Linda Welters, Colleen Callahan, Charlotte Jirousec, and Jane Farrell-Beck for their support and long-time interest.

Another person deserves special mention. During my graduate school days when I worked for him, Keith McFarland encouraged me, asked penetrating questions, sought clarification or simplification of my somewhat florid, non-academic writing, carefully and gently led me into safer paths of academic rhetoric, and generally mentored me for a future in academics. His support at a time when few really understood what I was trying to do meant more than I can possibly say. Two others from those days who helped frame who I became as a professor are Karal Ann Marling and Sarah Evans of the University of Minnesota. Each woman, outstanding in her own field, helped me through the mine fields of graduate school. Their inspiring teaching and wonderful writing opened my mind to worlds I had only imagined before. They taught me new ways to think, surely one of the greatest gifts of all.

I wish to thank Peggy Pinkerton for suggesting the title of this book. Another who deserves deepest thanks is Margaret Ewing. She has always encouraged me to think, even in the days when I was a stay-at-home mom. She has been my best critic, editor, and friend, and our recent paper published together (combining a costume historian and an aquatic ecologist) was the surprising professional outcome of a deep personal friendship and all those years of talking together—and it was exciting for both of us. She has been at the end of a phone for thirty years, and I am deeply grateful for her constancy and support.

Finally, my two sons, Geoffrey and Peter, have lived half their lives with their mother's involvement in this work, and probably have reached a point of disbelief that "the book" would ever see the light of day. For them, then, here it is.

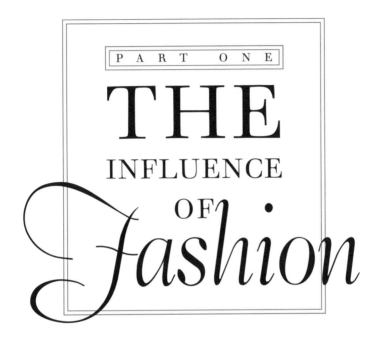

PART ONE

THE
INFLUENCE
OF
Fashion

PUBLIC CLOTHING
FOR
Outdoor Play

SPORT HAS MORE TO DO THAN ANYTHING ELSE WITH
THE EVOLUTION OF THE MODERN MODE; . . . THERE IS
ONLY ONE THING OF WHICH EVERYONE IS CONVINCED
. . . AND THAT IS THE PERFECTION OF THE ADAPTATION
TO THE NEEDS OF THE GAME WHICH MODERN DRESS
HAS EVOLVED.

British Vogue, *1926*

This book is about the origins of American sportswear, the most important clothing of the twentieth century and beyond. It is comfortable, easy, inexpensive, practical, and wearable by both men and women. It is undeniably American, yet it is worn by most people all over the world. We take it for granted. Yet this is the first time that such universality has existed in clothing, and it has lasted now for well over a half century—in itself a marvel, considering the speed of fashion change in this era of instant messages and images. Its pieces for women are readily understood and are so basic that they have lasted with very little fundamental change since the late 1920s: sweaters, pants, shirts, skirts, blazers. For men, the continuity in dress has lasted much longer, dating to the mid-nineteenth century. In fact, men's styles gave their look to women's. Yet up to World War II, without either preconception or reflection, clothing was sharply divided into men's wear on the one hand and women's on the other. There was no interest, it seemed, in finding common ground in dress. Both men and women were happy to dress appropriately for their sex, and were aghast when the bohemian few tried to cross over. Yet when the war came, all the conditions that had existed before vanished in the face of new need, new usage, and new attitudes about dress. After World War II, the pants and the easy, carefree pieces worn with them that women had donned during the war years were a permanent part of their wardrobes, and became the casual clothes they preferred, far from the elegant designer models and the polished Hollywood styles of the 1930s. Ever since then, although designers have kept alive the glamour of haute couture (indeed, in recent decades they have built an entire industry on glamorous showmanship and promotion rather than creativity), it is sportswear that fills the need, takes precedence, and has become the clothing of choice today.

Such enormous shifts of cultural understanding don't just happen overnight, even when projected into acceptance by something as devastating as a world war. Major upheavals had occurred before—the revolutionary wars of the eighteenth century and the Napoleonic wars of the early nineteenth come to mind—but even though they influenced dress, they never came close to bringing a change of such magnitude as came about in the twentieth century. For women to wear trousers, the symbol of masculinity for five hundred years, openly, acceptably, unthinkingly, accomplished what had never been done before in Western history. It gave women freedom in their dress, unbound from the societal and physical restrictions of the past. When we realize that only in the twentieth century did such a change in clothing occur, we have to ask, how did this happen? What created the conditions that World War II brought into focus?

The answer is the growing interest in sports and exercise that first came into public awareness some one hundred years before. It was sports that brought women out-of-doors into new activities that took them away from their housebound roles. It was sports that encouraged their latent competitive instincts. It was sports and exercise that changed their way of thinking about themselves. And when sport was mixed into the potent broth of higher education, the heady brew changed women, and certainly their clothing, forever.

Women's involvement in sports and exercise is a two-pronged history that begins in the early nineteenth century and ends a hundred years later when the two parts finally merge. The two parallel paths represent the wide range of games and sports that both men and women played together out-of-doors, and the exercises and gymnastics that eventually became known as physical education, performed by men and women separately, alone and generally indoors. When women first undertook these activities, they quite literally had nothing to wear. Over a period of decades, they cautiously devised new clothes for them, or modified the ones they had to serve the needs that active movement demanded. The breakthrough that shook off the restrictions of the Victorian age came with the new indoor sports of the 1890s, most specifically basketball for girls. From then on, comfort and common sense played an increasing role, finally overwhelming the conservatism and societal limitations that had kept women covered, compressed and usually in skirts. The result of the long, slow process is today's comfortable, practical clothing that the world recognizes as American sportswear.

Although the two types of activities for women developed at about the same time, each remained essentially separate from the other. Sport took place in the public sphere, exercise in the private. In public, women were expected to be modest and demure and to wear, to the best of their ability, the fashion of the time. Women's clothing for sport, then, was almost by definition clothing for interaction with men. Because it was social, fashion-oriented dress following the norms of the day, and worn out-of-doors in concept, it changed relatively slowly. It had to adhere to the constraints of "women's place" on women's behavior, including their clothing choices.

In contrast, the private sphere depended on the separation of the sexes, usually in an educational setting. Whereas young men had been educated together in their elite institutions for centuries, young women had not. It was a whole new idea to offer girls equal education. Therefore, this segregation of young women came into its own with the establishment of schools of higher learning for women. It was here, comfortably apart from the pressures of mixed-sex interaction, that clothing for physical education developed. It sprang from a burgeoning interest in exercise from the very beginning, with the founding of Mount Holyoke Seminary, later College, in the 1830s.[1] Unlike the clothing for sport, it was not hampered by the social constraints that operated when men were present. It depended instead on ideas of comfort and freedom of movement to guide its new forms. Both types of clothing took several decades to find their stride, but each had a separate origin and therefore evolved in a different way and at a different rate.

In Part One I tell the story of sport dress—public dress. This was the accepted clothing for women of the day, happily worn in mixed company, modified slightly for the new games and sports that emerged in the nineteenth century. Gymnastic dress, or private dress, will be dealt with in Part Two. But the double thrust—that is, activity undertaken with men on the one hand and single-sex activity within cloistered grounds on the other—together provided the seeds for the new ideas about clothing that took until the 1930s to come into full bloom. Only then, after each began borrowing from the other, did they merge indivisibly into the sensible, practical, and comfortable clothing of the twentieth century.

In simplest terms, the history of women's involvement in athletics in general and the foundations of sportswear in particular is in large measure the story of the long, slow adoption of trousers for women. It is a story that interweaves many different threads of a social history that has its beginnings in the eighteenth century. If trousers play an important role in this story, why, then, did women insist on retaining their fashionable outfits that included hats, gloves, corsets, crinolines, petticoats, and long full skirts as they eagerly participated in the many new games and activities that arose during the nineteenth century? Their look was calculated and unvarying—pert, active, and very, very feminine. The reason was simple. These were the clothes for courting. Sports represented a whole new arena for young men and women to meet and interact, usually for the first time without the eagle-eyed chaperon who had been a fixture of the past. And courting demanded the most attractive clothes one owned. In an age when marrying well was the goal of every woman, young ladies and young men too embraced with delight any new, socially acceptable way to engage with the opposite sex. Indeed, more often than not, a woman's entire future depended on marrying well since little else was open to her. No wonder, then, that "proper" clothing, that is, clothing that was both attractive and fashionable, became a significant consideration for both men and women as they participated in the new games and sports. The earliest of these were croquet and skating. Following hard on their heels came tennis, golf, swimming, and bicycling. All provided arenas for meeting and mating. The phenomenon of sport, any sport, as an opportunity for courting lasted through the century and well into the next. As an Outlook *magazine article from June 1899 titled "The Golfing Woman" put it, a man could learn as much in two hours in a mixed foursome as he could previously have learned in six weeks on a voyage with a prospective wife.[2]*

By the time that article was written at the end of the century, new outlets provided suitable settings and opportunities for members to meet and play games, mostly golf and tennis. The first American country club was established in Brookline, Massachusetts, in 1882, and soon every major city had one or more.[3] The country club appealed to families of similar background, offered a host of activities that brought young people together, and in the process encouraged a new version of class consciousness, even class structure in America.[4] Small wonder that fashionable clothing played a significant role.

But the clubs were not limited to the upper classes only. The growing middle classes, as represented by clerks or office workers and their peers, established clubs of their own at about the same time, usually for golf. The earliest of these in North America was the Montreal (later Royal Montreal) Golf Club, founded by an immigrant Scot, Alexander Dennistoun, in 1873. It is no surprise that the nineteenth-century invasion of Scots into Canada brought the game to the American continent, since the Royal and Ancient Game had been played in Scotland from at least the fifteenth century.[5] Soon after the Montreal club was founded, another appeared in Quebec City and still others in Ontario at Toronto, Brantford, Kingston, and Niagara. The first interprovincial matches between Ontario and Quebec were already being held by 1882, the same year that the Country Club of Brookline was opening its doors.[6]

The real boom for golf, though, came in the 1890s. The reasons were many, besides the growing population of Scots in North America. With the infusion of immigrants came new social and working conditions, each of which touched on the rising interest in sports. The newcomers settled not in the farmlands that had lured their predecessors but rather in the cities, feeding the burgeoning urban population at the end of the century. The influx of newcomers changed the nature of work at this time as well. The sheer volume of immigrants, combined with a new awareness of working conditions, led to reform in the guise of a shorter work week. With increased leisure time came the growing desire for more leisure activities. In addition, the improvement of public transportation solved the problem of getting to the major sites of leisure activity, whether the beach or tennis courts or golf links. Interestingly, perhaps the greatest influence on the rising popularity of golf in the 1890s was the bicycle. It, possibly more than any other single innovation, eased the restrictions that had hampered the middle-class Victorian woman. It gave her a new, simple, and relatively inexpensive form of transportation and offered her freedom as well. Simultaneously, a "tremendous number of women" took up golf in the 1890s. They even formed their own clubs: the first, again, in Montreal with another in Toronto in 1891. Women "joined in droves."[7]

9

Clearly, then, the activities and expectations that were in place by the beginning of the twentieth century had broadened tremendously over the preceding few decades. And the dress the participants wore cannot be ignored. This section on "public clothing," then, will reveal its close relationship to fashion wear, with its mere nod to the demands of active movement. To track this history, I look at the most influential sports: tennis, swimming, and bicycling. But I begin with croquet and skating, since these two represented the introduction of women into sporting activities. Golf, though an important new sport in the 1890s, failed to generate new ideas in clothing (and in fact has remained heroically staid as far as dress is concerned throughout the entire ensuing century) so will not be a part of this study. Neither will riding and the equestrian sports, which have a tradition of their own, founded primarily on upper-class lifestyles.[8] As golf clothing remained outside the trends that propelled the change in clothing for other sports, so too did riding gear. After about 1910 to 1915, jodhpurs, hacking jacket, and splendid boots became codified as the uniform of choice for men and women riders alike. At the beginning of the twenty-first century, riding dress tradition remains intact, based now on a style that is almost a century old. These sports are the exceptions. As for all the rest, the American middle class wholeheartedly embraced them with joy and fervor. Each presented its own set of problems in the matter of dress.

The clothing of any period reflects its cultural environment. To appreciate how long this journey has been, we must understand the societal factors that led to the acceptance of sports in the first place.

FACTORS
OF
Change

As with most movements that revolutionize a nation, the impulses that led to the sports craze of the nineteenth century came from many different sources rather than developing in a clear, linear fashion. As for the clothing that was deemed suitable for the new activities, we have seen that there were decided societal reasons for it to remain closely tied in style and form to the fashions of the period. The clothes themselves, as all clothes do, sprang from the circumstances and the mood of the time and reflected the dominant cultural environment, so it is to those we must turn. Studying the clothing lets us study the period.

Throughout the twentieth century, scholars and commentators wrote about the rise of the middle class and about the subsequent rise in the notions of leisure and recreation. The shift away from the eighteenth century's practices of democracy and partnership between men and women to the nineteenth century's recognition of "women's role" polarized the sexes into separate spheres of public and private. Men, of course, were "public," and women were "private." In tandem with the development of this concept was the growth of leisure time and the ways in which it was spent by each sex. Visitors to the United States in the 1830s and 1840s frequently reported a doleful lack of amusements or indeed any form of activity other than moneymaking among the men they met in their travels throughout the country. Even then they could readily identify the upward mobility, the overwork, and the constant push towards financial success that has become so typical of American life, so much a part of the American character. And though they may seem strange bedfellows, this concern for money existed hand in hand with a sturdy revivalist religion that puritanically denounced any sort of pleasure. With this combination generating a national mood, the "new" pastimes had an uphill battle. The famous preacher Henry Ward Beecher, member of the great New England Beecher family and brother of Catharine Beecher and Harriet Beecher Stowe, helped lead the charge. In 1844 he vilified the theater, the concert hall, and the circus, promising everlasting damnation to any who partook of the siren charms of those benign amusements.[1] This repressed New England viewpoint was shared in many other parts of the country. It was not until the growing middle class came to realize that the evangelists were actually pandering to a narrow segment of the population that people began to recognize that simple pleasures might after all be both healthy and morally acceptable.[2]

Many other factors helped bring about the great changes the United States underwent during the first half of the nineteenth century. Not least of these was the urbanization of America, which in turn affected sports. The influx of immigrants certainly helped to build and democratize private clubs for golf and other sports at the end of the century, but even in the early years the changes were significant. Between 1800 and 1850, the population living in urban centers of eight thousand or more tripled. Of course, in comparison to the astonishing growth of the late nineteenth century, these numbers were small. But they were sufficently impressive to bring to light the emerging problems of crowding and the lack of opportunities for leisure pastimes that existed in America's cities. As one foreign visitor, Michael Chevalier, somewhat patronizingly observed in 1833: "Democracy is too new a comer upon the earth to have been able as yet to organize its pleasures and amusements. In Europe, our pleasures are essentially exclusive, they are aristocratic like Europe itself. In this matter, then, as in politics, the American democracy has yet to create every thing fresh."[3] Slowly, however, America did just that. Its response was a gradual introduction of the commercial amusements that would ultimately explode into the vast entertainment industry we know today. By and large, though, organized sports did not find their way into the American social fabric until after the Civil War.[4]

Not all of the innovations were directed towards play. The United States in the mid-nineteenth century was ripe for an explosion in the cultural arena as well. Here the money, leisure time, and earnest attention were focused instead on elevating the gentility of the population at large. As John F. Kasson stated in his history of leisure activity in America, *Amusing the Millions*, "a self-conscious elite of critics, ministers, educators, and reformers" living primarily in the urban Northeast flowed into the vacuum to assume cultural leadership. These "genteel reformers" sought to instruct the turbulent and rough-edged democracy, to bring to it a semblance of refinement and discipline. The "American apostles of culture" strenuously labored to inculcate the Victorian virtues of "character—moral integrity, self-control, sober earnestness, industriousness—among the citizenry at large." Their seriousness of purpose dictated that all activities, whether work or leisure, were to be constructive. In the process, they legitimized poetry, fiction, the visual arts, serious music, and other cultural pursuits, not "for art's sake" but, in Kasson's words, "for their moral and social utility." Their work in turn inspired those who followed them to endow the nation with the museums, art galleries, libraries, symphony orchestras, and other institutions that set the tone and the cultural goals for the century to come, in terms of both quality and philanthropy. Indeed, only in the past decade or so has the 150-year-old mold been broken, as cultural institutions are moving away from the paternalistic goals they represented towards a more truly recognizable democratic focus.[5]

The rise of the genteel reformers intersected in three ways with the rise of sports and athletic activity for women. The first was through their farsighted donations of land to develop urban parks, to create peaceful green areas for the otherwise city-bound. The second, which will be discussed in Part Two, was to found colleges for women. The third, which took a slightly different shape from the other two because it was promoted by women, for women, was the dress reform movement. It will be discussed briefly in chapter 6.

Of course, the idea of greens and commons was not new to nineteenth-century America. These had been an integral part of colonial towns from the beginning. But the first planned public park, designed to enhance nature and to counteract the relentless pressure of an overcrowded commercial environment, was New York's Central Park. Frederick Law Olmsted, little known at that time, submitted a design with architect Calvert

Vaux. They placed first in the 1858 competition. Olmsted was put in charge of the project. It was so successful and so widely admired that it inspired the creation of many city parks around the country. Olmsted worked on most of the similar projects in America, among them Prospect Park in Brooklyn; Fairmount Park in Philadelphia; South Park in Chicago; River-side and Morningside Parks, also in New York City; Mount Royal Park in Montreal; the Capitol grounds in Washington, D.C.; the park system of Buffalo, New York; the "Emerald Necklace" linking the Boston Common and the Public Garden with the Fenway and other greenways along the Charles River; and the campus of Stanford University in Palo Alto. He is regarded as the father of American landscape architecture.[6]

In Central Park, Olmsted sought to meld a democratic recreational set-ting with "an artfully natural landscape." He planned for horseback riding, boating on the pond in the summer, and skating in the winter. But he was careful to keep the louder and rougher, more boisterous sports and games of the working class out of his park. A true representative of his gentleman class, he wanted his park to project instead a calming, restorative interac-tion with nature. Central Park was popular in spite of its uptown location, which required considerable planning and expenditure for most people to get there. Statistics bear this out: in 1871 an average of 30,000 people vis-ited it every day, for a total of 10 million over the entire year.[7] This was at a time when the population of the city stood at 942,000, and of the entire state of New York at 4.382 million.[8] Clearly, the park was an idea whose time had come, the first of many throughout the country.

At the same time that green areas were being developed to give urban dwellers a place to escape and to pursue healthier living, several influential groups were becoming aware of what they regarded as the general unhealthiness of middle-class American women. These complaints ranged widely, from sources as varied as the vocal foreigners who came to America and criticized what they found, to educators such as Catharine Beecher, to medical practitioners, among them the pioneering women in the field. Among the targets of their attacks were the various "cures" of the time, including the popular water cures that Beecher, for one, periodically indulged in, or the rest cure that kept a woman flat on her back, immobile, for as much as six weeks at a time to rid her of "hysteria." It began to dawn on the critics as they recognized the drawbacks of these cures that, by contrast, gentle exercise might actually be beneficial to good health.[9]

At just about this time the medical profession had fallen into disrepute, with justifiable cause. Standards of schooling in many cases were minimal at best, and either scarcely addressed or entirely ignored basic scientific knowledge. A case in point was the Geneva Medical College, where Elizabeth Blackwell, the first woman in America to be trained as a doctor, received her education. It had been founded in 1835, and by 1847, the year of Blackwell's entry, had seven faculty.[10] A medical degree there required two sixteen-week courses of lectures (two semesters of work, by today's standards), a thesis, and an oral exam to graduate. Granted, each student had to have some background in science and classical languages, at that time taught only to young men in schools, and some prior medical experience upon entry—though under the circumstances, one wonders where they were to get it. Even so, although the requirements seem woefully meager by today's standards, they were enough to keep women out of the profession. Blackwell's prior education lacked all the pre-admission requirements, and so she was forced to learn the science and languages on her own. In addition, she spent a year living in the home of a sympathetic doctor, who gave her access to his medical books and to the breadth of his knowledge. Her road was not an easy one. Even though she became a favorite at the school and graduated first in her class, the initial reaction to her was hostile and remained uneasy throughout her stay. Indeed, after she graduated, the dean of the college stated that although he personally admired her very much, the "inconvenience attending the admission of all qualified females" was so great that he was "compelled on all future occasions to oppose such a practice."

Perhaps because of her own ordeal while being trained alongside men and then striving to be recognized in the profession, or perhaps simply because she was a woman of her time, Blackwell was ever mindful of the decorum that existed between the sexes. But precisely because it was "unnatural" for women patients "to have no resort but to men" in those diseases "peculiar to themselves . . . no woman of sensibility" could allow herself to be examined by a male physician "without great reluctance."[11] She therefore encouraged other women to come into the field. Dr. Ann Preston agreed. In 1851 she was one of eight members of the first graduating class (and later the dean) of the Women's Medical College of Pennsylvania in Philadelphia, which had been founded by male Quakers the year before. She too believed that teaching women medicine was "a step not *from* but *towards* decency and decorum."[12] Before long, not only medical schools but teaching hospitals as well were founded by women, for women, as Blackwell and her followers broke down the barriers, bringing a new awareness of women's concerns into medical practice, not just in the United States but in Great Britain, too. *Godey's Lady's Book*, ever proud of the women who were among its readers, reported in 1866:

> We do things better in America. Medical colleges for women have been founded here during the last fifteen years; there are, probably, from three to four hundred graduates, who hold the full degree of "Doctress of Medicine," now in successful practice in our Republic. Here is the announcement of the one *British Doctress:*——
>
> "Miss Elizabeth Garrett has passed her final examination at Apothecaries' Hall, London, and received a license as a general practitioner of medicine. This is the first instance that has occurred in England, but several other ladies are pursuing their medical studies, and there is a growing feeling among medical men, as well as among the general public, in favor of women practitioners. It is admitted here that to Philadelphia is due the credit of first inaugurating this movement."[13]

Blackwell herself, though, perhaps with a certain sense of inevitability but more likely a deep and compelling desire to work with needy women, turned from the male area of "doctoring" to the promotion of hygiene and what was then termed physical education—literally, education about the body and its health and well-being. With this, she directed her attention to an area that was virtually ignored at the time, the public health needs of the urban poor. As part of her effort, she published a series of "Lectures on the Laws of Life" in 1852, arguing the need for "physical education" and exercise.[14] Interestingly, she tied the body to its clothing, in a sense foreshadowing the developments of the late twentieth century: "We need developed muscles that shall make the human body really a divine image, a perfect form rendering all dress graceful, and not requiring to be patched and filled up and weighed down with clumsy contrivances for hiding its deformities."[15] She also was an early advocate of "equally balanced bodies, minds, hearts and souls,"[16] later reshaped into the clarion call for a sound mind in a sound body, *mens sana in corpore sano.*

Parenthetically, as sexual barriers were being broken, so were color barriers. One of the early medical pioneers was Rebecca J. Cole, the first African American physician in the United States, who graduated in 1867 from the Women's Medical College of Pennsylvania. She spent the years 1872 to 1881 as a resident physician at the New York Infirmary for Women and Children, a hospital owned and operated by women physicians, and later worked with Blackwell as a "sanitary visitor," a traveling physician who visited slum families in their homes and instructed them in family hygiene and prenatal and infant care.[17] By the 1870s and 1880s, in the post–Civil War years, women were increasingly being trained as doctors in schools such as Philadelphia's.[18] Nevertheless, the control of the profession remained firmly in men's hands.

Despite women's entry into the medical field, it was the overall failure to cure that led to the rise of the health reform movement. Stimulated in part by the few women in medicine, but even more so by men and women outside the medical profession who wished to educate the population about the virtues of a healthful diet, public hygiene, and physical exercise, as well as basic physiology (the "physical education" addressed in Blackwell's tract), it developed quite separately from the mainstream medical profession. Many of the women active in these groups were women's rights advocates and dress reformers.[19] Their desire to lift the veil of ignorance from Victorian women by teaching them about their own bodies was a radical notion, but it became increasingly widespread. Articles on health and hygiene, women's education in general, and women's medical education in particular, appeared in the popular press. For example, a single 1864 issue of the influential *Godey's Lady's Book* reported "Vassar College To Be Opened This Year!"; advocated "Free National Normal Schools For Young Women"; and discussed "The Medical Profession: What Women Have Done In It."[20] But even as *Godey's*, in the person of Sarah Josepha Hale, advocated medical training for women, it was careful to maintain Victorian propriety. In a July article from that same year, we finally glimpse the social constraints and expectations for women, even if seen through the eyes of an ardent supporter:

> We hope, for the honor of our sex, that these gentle *M.D.'s* will insist on retaining their womanhood in their profession, and never assume the style and title of man as *Doctor*, when their own *Doctress* is better and more elegant, being delicate, definite, and dignified.... We do not want *female* physicians, that compound term signifying an *animal man*; we want cultivated, refined feminine physicians, known as *Doctresses* for their own sex and children, and conservers of domestic health and happiness....
>
> One truth is sure; a lady can never elevate herself by becoming manlike or making pretenses to be so. She must keep her own place, cultivate her own garden of home.[21]

Fortunately for women's health, even some of the male leaders in the medical profession, such as S. Weir Mitchell, the quintessential Victorian doctor, joined in the demand for more exercise for women. "To run, to climb, to swim, to ride, to play violent games, ought to be as natural to the girl as to the boy."[22] Or, in Mrs. Hale's florid prose, "I can see before me a long line of puny, sickly children that have been recommended by physicians to the exercise of gymnastics, in order to restore health and vigor to their feeble frames."[23]

With mention of *Godey's*, it is time to consider another factor that changed the countenance of America—the popular press. Many historians have commented on its enormous impact from the early nineteenth century on in influencing the growth of trends, fads, and passions in the United States.[24] Advances in technology created new presses that improved both printing and engraving, and developed a new kind of paper, made from wood rather than rags. These inventions cut costs in the process, yielding a cheap product available to everybody, as with, for example, the "pulps" of the end of the century. Artists leaped to the task of capturing American life in their illustrations, sending swift visual messages across the country with the help of a burgeoning railway system, helping to draw together the vast expanses with their sparse but growing settlements. The twenty-two-year-old Winslow Homer was one of these illustrators, projecting the spirit of mid-century America when he began working for *Harper's Weekly* in 1857. His graphic representations, a feature of the magazine until 1875, gave his generation views of everything from skating in a still-barren Central Park in 1860 to Civil War battles in Virginia, to bathing at Newport.[25] For the first time, then, a communications medium showed its power to disseminate fashion, trends, and events.

Women provided a new and rapidly growing readership—what today we would call a target audience—for the barrage of magazines created to address all aspects of their daily lives and interests. For the first time, because of a new broader literacy, women formed a vital, even avid audience for the swelling numbers of female authors, many of whom wrote not just for the new magazines but books, too, that resonated with the morality of the day. Indeed, these authors, through magazines such as *Godey's*, helped to establish the parameters of women's sphere.

The Industrial Revolution had jolted society out of its comfortable pastoral quietude. As we have seen, stunning changes followed in its wake: technological advances, a burgeoning urban population and its attendant problems, new kinds of wealth and a distinctive leisure class, and mass production, to name a few. Hand in hand with this last came the department store. It provided a new kind of outlet for the manufactured goods, often textile products, that attempted to satisfy the demands of the moneyed and leisured. The sewing machine made it all possible.

The idea for a sewing machine had been around since the late eighteenth century, but most attempts to produce one had failed. The key to success came only when inventors broke away from trying to imitate traditional hand-sewing methods and introduced two completely innovative concepts: a new type of needle and a double, looped thread combination. Baltasar Krems of Mayern, Germany, provided the first in 1810. His crank-operated chain stitch machine for sewing nightcaps had a continuous material feed and, significantly, a needle with the eye at its point. A series of tinkerers and inventors continued to tackle the problem in the early nineteenth century. Among the more successful was the French tailor Barthelemy Thimonnier, in 1830. Alas, his success was also his downfall. Traditional tailors, afraid for their livelihood, attacked and destroyed his eighty-machine factory, forcing him to escape with his life. Four years later, Walter Hunt built America's first sewing machine but, fearing that his invention would destroy jobs, backed away. It was Elias Howe, working in Boston for a man who repaired precision instruments, who hit on the process of using two threads from different sources: a Krems-style needle with its eye at the point pushed through the cloth to form a loop on the underside that was anchored by another thread slipped through the loop with a shuttle, to create the lock stitch. He received a patent in 1846, but his machine cost $300, more than any householder could easily afford.[26] A series of disasters followed, and bad business moves hampered his progress and his ultimate financial success.

Even though Howe never made a success of his invention, the sewing machine business took off. By the 1850s, many manufacturers had stolen his idea, and found eager sewers to use their machines. The best of these was designed by Isaac Merritt Singer, a flamboyant actor, machinist, and ladies' man whose genius lay more in marketing than in invention. Singer's was the first really practical sewing machine; as long as it had thread, it sewed and maintained an even and balanced stitch on both the right and wrong sides. Patented in 1851, Singer's machine kept Howe's lock stitch process and needle but it improved the ease of use. It did away with Howe's old hand crank in favor of a treadle and used a "perpendicular action" (it was marketed under the name Perpendicular Action Sewing Machine) in which the needle moved up and down rather than sideways. Its patent claims were threefold: it regulated the cloth feed, it controlled the tension on the needle thread, and it lubricated the needle thread to allow it to sew leather. Its main claim to fame, though, apart from the relief it gave women who had been chained to unending hand-sewing, was that it was the first domestic appliance to be mass-manufactured on an assembly line, using interchangeable parts. As a result, the Singer sewing machines could be produced in quantity and sold for a much lower price than earlier models.

With this innovation, marketing followed. Singer introduced several techniques that are still in use today, now so much a part of our modern way of doing business that we never stop to wonder where they began. Singer, the unfailing ladies' man, was the first to display his product in a well-appointed showroom, using comely young women to demonstrate the machine. They taught buyers how to operate them as well. He devised the installment plan, five dollars down and the remainder, with interest, in monthly payments. He offered half-price deals to church sewing circles, which would buy one machine for the group—a brilliant double play that lent respectability to his machine as it built up individual appetites among the members, who would each want her own. And he offered a fifty-dollar buy-back on an old machine to anyone buying a new one.[27] *Godey's* gave its stamp of approval in February 1863: "The benefits of this wonderful invention increase with every year of its trial. . . . The Sewing-Machine comes into the heart of the home; it helps in the domestic circle; it has an important influence on family comfort and social happiness."[28] The next month, as if to seal the blessing, a charming engraving, "The New Sewing Machine," portrayed two beautifully dressed young ladies seated in the parlor using their machine, with a copy of *Godey's* open on a stool beside it.[29]

This marvelous machine was to revolutionize the manufacture of clothing. By the late 1850s, the *New York News* pointed out that "men are not only being fed, and transported from point to point by the aid of machinery, but they are also clothed by it. The increasing millions of civilized men and women are no longer exclusively dependent for comfort and tasteful garments upon the slow operations of mere manual labor." By the mid-1850s, the sewing machine provided the backbone for the ready-made clothing industry, manufacturing shirts, collars, and other furnishings. And for women, in a miracle of timing that one suspects was causal rather than coincidental, the necessary crinolines and hoops of the later 1850s and 1860s, both hard to sew by hand, became much easier to produce with the sewing machine.[30]

All these developments notwithstanding, the idea of mass-manufacturing clothing in America was not new. It had begun with army uniforms during the War of 1812, though this had been accomplished by coordinating hand-sewers. The sewing machine took over that role with the demands of the Civil War. The Union Army needed over 1.5 million uniforms a year; the sewing machine answered the call and demonstrated to a postwar industry what could be accomplished. Happily, or, more likely, even because of the speedy construction the sewing machine allowed, men's styles in the 1850s introduced a new relaxed fit and a simpler line. The lounge or sack jacket, precursor to the modern-day suit, straight-cut and clean in line, required far less tailoring to the body, and therefore lent itself more easily to mass production and ready-to-wear than older styles. In the post–Civil War years, for the same reasons, women's outerwear (cloaks, wraps, and the wide-skirted semi-coat styles of mid-century) as well as underwear (hoops, drawers and petticoats) were also machine-made and sold in retail stores, in particular the department store, which had emerged from its more tentative beginnings in the 1850s.

Many of the great retail establishments opened in the 1850s and 1860s: Jordan Marsh in Boston (1851); Marshall Field's (1852) and Carson Pirie Scott (1854) in Chicago; Macy's (1858) and A. T. Stewart's (1861) in New York; John Wanamaker's in Philadelphia (1862). The majority of them directly and deliberately targeted the growing company of middle-class customers with discretionary money to spend, rather than appealing to the working class, who came mainly to rub shoulders and look. The idea of the department store grew out of the older general stores as well as the new specialty shops that catered to women. The 1870s saw the introduction of almost every service that a twentieth-century department store shopper would come to expect: refreshment facilities, whether a soda fountain, a lunch counter, or a lady's luncheon court or tearoom; ladies' lounges complete with comfortable chairs, even writing desks with stationery and newspapers; sparkling lavatories; delivery service; and, by the 1880s, even telephone and telegraph stations, lost and founds, post offices, and other services. Macy's and Wanamaker's had electric lights as well by the late 1870s. Catalogue shopping was first introduced by Montgomery Ward in 1872, made possible by the expanding web of railroads that now linked the country. The only thing lacking was the charge account, a twentieth-century lure. Even the "event" sales and specials so familiar to today's shoppers were in place by the late 1880s: seasonal clearances and events for Christmas, Valentine's Day, and the like spurred sales. Early on, the stores learned the draw of special programming. In 1887, for example, Wanamaker's hosted a period costume extravaganza, complete with an 1880s version of 1780s styles, to celebrate the centennial of the U.S. Constitution. And, in the spirit of the day, capitalizing on the infatuation for sports, Macy's held an archery contest. The success was stunning: within just five years after the Civil War, in 1870, Macy's sales totaled over $1 million and continued to rise by 80 percent each of the next seven years. Thus the selling of goods became a partnership with the selling of class, of trendy activities, even of sports. [31]

Although women's clothing was slower to be mass-produced than men's, by the 1870s much of women's requisite (and plentiful) underwear was factory-made and available both in stores and by mail order. By 1887, Jordan Marsh took note of this: "Only a few years ago, [ready-made clothing] was in its infancy; and what then was a spasmodic beginning is now a giant enterprise."[32] The process was slow but steady, helped in great measure by the introduction of Montgomery Ward's catalogue and others that followed, including those of the T. Eaton Company, centered in Toronto, whose earliest catalogue dated to 1881, and Sears Roebuck, which entered the catalogue business in 1888. By century's end, clothing not only could be made in quantity, it could be shipped in quantity anywhere in the United States and Canada. With a central source of dissemination of goods advertised widely through the ever-expanding print media, manufacturers and designers had stronger and more immediate control over what the country would wear.

All these interwoven factors, together with the broader availability and tolerance of higher education for women, helped set the scene for the acceptance of sports and exercise for women. Advances in technology changed not just the manufacture and merchandising of clothing but the textiles used in it. Not only could a huge quantity of cloth be turned out, dropping prices considerably, but also new kinds of machine-made cloth appeared. Knitting machines introduced a more flexible textile that "gave" on the body when it was in motion. Called "jersey," it was adopted for tennis dress as early as 1879.[33] And with the growth of the sport movement, the demand for suitable clothing—*fashionable* suitable clothing—grew too.

The technical advances of the Industrial Revolution also encouraged the production and distribution of more sophisticated and cheaper sports equipment to a wider audience—often through the catalogues. As we will see with the bicycle, these goods stimulated a universal craze that swept the land, gathering all segments of society in every part of the United States and Canada.

WOMEN MOVE
Out-of-$Doors$

Croquet and Skating

A WIDELY ADMIRED FASHION THEORY STATES THAT MANY SOCIETAL SHIFTS are introduced by the upper classes and "trickle down" to those lesser mortals striving to rise to their level. To complete the cycle, when the fashion leaders see what they have wrought they hastily abandon it and move on to the next great enthusiasm.[1] Time and again, writers have claimed the truth of this when speaking of croquet, tennis, bicycling, even baseball. By and large, they claim, these pastimes were borrowed from English games and played, as no one would question, by the British upper classes. But a look at the introduction of games and sports into the United States reveals an American twist to the story which reflects the singularly independent character of the American people. Here, the "common" people enjoyed their games and amusements perhaps even more than their social superiors did. Mid-century visitors to the United States reported that the Americans they met took little or no exercise of any kind. Significantly, those Americans were mainly members of the leisured class, not the average working man, who, it would seem, never crossed paths with the observant visitors.

What we would now call spectator sports also emerged in the nineteenth century—everything from upper-class sailing regattas to much more democratic activities ranging from horse racing to cockfights and shell games. As one visitor commented in his diary however, although "there were a great many people here, male and female, . . . in my opinion [there were] few respectable ones."[2] It was the working class, not the elite, who actually participated in "the boisterous fun and rough sports" that Olmsted tried so hard to keep out of Central Park. In addition, immigrants had brought their masculine gymnastics and sports with them from their native countries. The Germans, for example, organized the first *Turnverein*, or gymnastic society, in the United States, in Cincinnati in 1848. By the outbreak of the Civil War, there were 157 societies in 27 states.[3] The Caledonian Games of the Scots, forerunners of the track-and-field competitions of a later date, met first in Boston in 1853, then Hoboken, New Jersey, in 1857.[4] In a nice reversal of the trickle-down theory, native-born Americans had played pickup games such as "town ball" or rounders (English children's games, it must be admitted) since the eighteenth century. It was these that provided the basis for baseball, whose rules were changed and formalized by New York's Knickerbocker Base Ball Club in the mid-century years following the first meeting of the Knickerbockers and the New York Nines at Elysian Fields in Hoboken on June 19, 1846.[5]

One might say, then, that the Anglo-Saxon love of games and sports formed a distinct part of the American character. This devotion was carried on the shoulders of the common man into the nineteenth century, when it was reinforced by the first waves of immigrants to this country. But because genteel society—the rapidly expanding middle class—of the 1830s, 1840s, and 1850s regarded it as unfashionable (not to say uncouth) to play sports, it took a societal revolution of sorts to make them acceptable on a nationwide basis. And perhaps the opening shots of the revolution were fired on that selfsame field in Hoboken by the upper-class Knickerbockers, with their code of "base ball." By the 1850s, other more democratic clubs had appeared, clubs of workers (shipwrights, mechanics, truckmen), forcing the Knickerbockers to accept the fact that "the great mass, who are in a subordinate capacity can participate in this health giving and noble pastime." After all, the only necessities of the game were a bat, a ball, and a place to play.[6]

Although the United States immediately prior to the Civil War was on the brink of the sports explosion that still engulfs American society today, the phenomenon was single-sexed. It took a gentler, more refined pastime, one more reflective of the idealized woman of mid-century America, to encourage women to participate in any outdoor activity. That pastime was croquet.

It has been said that croquet brought women outdoors. In truth, two activities accomplished that. The other, as we shall see, was skating. Croquet, though, was the first game that lured young women out to play with men. Before that, according to an 1865 croquet rule book, women's opportunities had been scant indeed: "Hitherto, while men and boys have had their healthful means of recreation in the open air, the women and girls have been restricted to the less exhilarating sports of indoor life; or, if they adventure out, all the participation in the healthful outdoor amusement and exercise they could indulge in was the tame and unsatisfactory position of mere lookers-on."[7]

Croquet's history is murky. It is thought to have come from a medieval French peasant game called *paille maille* that was brought to the English court of Charles II in the seventeenth century.[8] Its later rebirth in England came sometime around 1852 or 1853 in an 1830s Irish game called crooky. Croquet, as it became more genteelly known, began as an aristocratic pastime played on the wide, well-groomed lawns of the rich. That soon changed. As a possible explanation, its appearance at the same time as the invention and manufacture of the reel lawn mower is a coincidence too great to ignore. A Gloucestershire man, Edwin Beard Budding, produced the first lawn mower in the 1830s, but after his patents ran out in the mid-1850s, many versions of the machine were available. At about that time, croquet as a game democratized.[9]

Within the first year or so after its introduction into England, an English toy maker, John Jaques, began to mass-produce the equipment. Even though he used expensive basswood in order to charge high prices, he found a booming and eager market. America followed hard behind, copying the Jaques designs. Very quickly croquet adapted to smaller, rougher lawns and public parks, undoubtedly by now being mowed by machine rather than by animal.

The most widely recognized contemporary representations of croquet players are Winslow Homer's, dating from 1865 to 1869, just as the game's popularity was peaking. His paintings show middle-class Americans, one of them a first cousin of Homer's, playing on wide, long-shadowed, green late-afternoon lawns during the time of day preferred by most players. Women dominate all five of the paintings. In this, Homer reflected the reality of the game. The writers and reporters of the time repeatedly commented that croquet was the first sport to allow women to participate in a

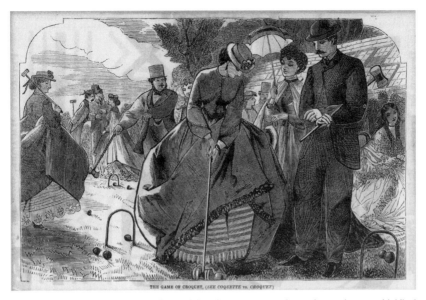

THE GAME OF CROQUET, (SEE *COQUETTE* vs. *CROQUET*)

"The Game of Croquet," about 1867. The social setting, party atmosphere, elegant dresses with hiked skirts that display decorative petticoats, and concentration on the game are evident. Collection of the author.

physical activity in the company of men. Because of this, croquet parties were incorporated into other social activities that women organized during the summer season—weekend parties, lavish champagne suppers, dinner parties, and dances. A colored fashion plate from *Peterson's Magazine* in July 1870 portrays "a lawn party, with croquet players, etc., etc. These parties are going to be very fashionable, this summer, in the country," declares the commentary. "They are given in the daytime, and out-of-doors, though, sometimes, they finish with a dance, in-doors, after sunset."[10]

As croquet's appeal spread, and with the publication of a spate of books that gave not only the rules of the game but rules of gracious conduct as well, women seemed to have taken over. At that point, a new woman emerged. The game's critical moment came with "the croquet," when the player who has the advantage over her opponent lines up her ball with his, places her foot on her own ball, swings her mallet, and smacks his ball "off to China"—not a gentle, submissive, feminine play by any means. Women were enjoined to be both graceful and ladylike during the game, but they were illustrated over and over performing precisely this aggressive—and aggravating—croquet move, and appearing to enjoy themselves as they did. Clearly, croquet opened new worlds for women, including the newly visible outlets of sexuality and competitiveness.

As they seemingly ponder their next moves, Homer's thoughtful croquet players are dressed in the height of fashion. They wear hoops and crino-lines, their outer skirts hitched up with an "elevator" device to display the intricate detailing of the underskirts.[11] With any luck for the opponents or spectators, this might allow a glimpse of an alluring foot and ankle during the dreaded "croquet" play. Their tiny waists are emphasized with belts, their white sleeves crisp and full, enhanced by shawls or a trim sleeveless bolero. Pert hats, beribboned and befeathered, tilt over their brows, shading their eyes, and their hands are protected in elegant leather gloves as they clutch or swing their mallets. This might be garden party attire; indeed, it probably was. It certainly looks like the clothing of attraction.

The croquet lawn became famous as a meeting ground for young eligi-bles, as a socially acceptable place to carry on flirtations. Indeed, so well understood was this benefit of the game that authors referred to it again and again. Sexual innuendo peppered contemporary accounts, and croquet became synonymous with man-hunting. One popular witticism archly declared, "She, whom he came to croquet, croquets him," while another, even bolder, claimed that "croquet may to Hymen's Alter lead." Perhaps this, more than anything else, explains its wild popularity in the 1860s and 1870s. An English advocate of the game, clearly aware of the proliferation of gambling that was a part of almost all male sports and pastimes of the era, stated, "Perhaps the finest argument in favor of croquet. . . is its moral-ity. It has no taint attached to it, and never will. It is too refined. . .ever to become a gambler's game."[12] Perhaps so, since it had rapidly become iden-tified as a female-oriented pastime. But the problem lay, rather, in the "contact and competition between the sexes. . . sublimated into an elegant, highly formalized ritual, occurring in a deceptively wholesome garden set-ting, amidst a display of finery and manners. . . . Fashion set the tone for gentle titillation." In seeming support of this, in 1868 *Harper's Bazar* called croquet "an exquisite game, at which the stakes are soft glances and wreathing smiles, and where hearts are lost and won."[13]

Here, the proper clothing certainly played its role. The hoop skirt, espe-cially one hiked up for the game, directed attention to the foot, positioned to "croquet" the ball.[14] Tiny feet were the hallmark of beauty. Feet and ankles became erotic areas of the female body during this period, possibly because they were visible for the first time in generations. "Now that the decree has gone forth in favor of short dresses," declared *Godey's Lady's Book* in 1867, "we must look to our boots. As harmony of color prevails to a great extent in dress, boots and shoes should also accord."[15] This edict presented a problem in playing croquet. Women were warned against wearing white shoes as being impractical even though perfect for summer wear, and indeed one can imagine the chagrin on discovering one's best white shoes all grass-stained for the duration of the season. But players eventually found solutions for the difficulty, thanks to the vulcanization of rubber, a process developed earlier in the century. Waterproof boots were invented in the United States as early as the 1820s, and Wait Webster of New York registered a patent for attaching india-rubber soles in 1832.[16] It took another thirty-five years and the immense popularity of croquet to create the demand for the first kind of sneaker—indeed, the first shoe specifically designed for sport—in the form of a laced canvas upper with a rubber sole. It was American by manufacture and was called a "croquet sandal."[17] Later improvements in rubber processing spawned rubbers that slipped over the shoes. By 1886, Bloomingdale's was advertising a slip-on pump called "Ladies Croquets," with a pair of rubbers available in the same style, made out of "extra light weight gossamer" rubber.[18]

Overall, though, dressing appropriately for the active and lively outdoor game of croquet was a minor consideration. Devotees preferred to dress attractively. A rule book from 1865 scolded: "With all deference, we suggest to all ladies that, where it is possible, they should dress with some regard to the requirements of the game; it is hardly conducive to elegance to behold a half dozen officious gentlemen hovering about a lady as train-bearers and flycatchers whenever she wishes to perform the croquet, and we protest against those sweeping skirts that whisk the balls about and change the whole feature of the field."

Those sweeping skirts posed other problems as well. The stroke called "spooning" was a pendulum swing of the mallet, executed between the legs. Ladies could not perform it but had to side-swing across in front of them instead. "We agree that spooning is perfectly fair in a match of gentlemen, but it is decidedly ungenerous when played with ladies, unless those ladies are bloomers," declared *The Nation* in the mid-1860s.[19] As we will see in Part Two, only an intrepid, not to say scandalous, few were "bloomers" in the 1860s.

In spite of the difficulties the clothing of the day presented to the gentle players of the challenging and exciting, even sexual game of croquet, they wore it without question. They offered their most appealing toilette, calculated as carefully as their next croquet move. Their futures depended on it. And besides, there was no other acceptable alternative to wear in genteel mixed company.

What croquet was to summertime, skating was to winter. It had become an increasingly alluring pastime during the late 1850s and 1860s but took a little while to catch on for women. Magazines of the time played their role in popularizing it. Once again, we turn to Winslow Homer and the double-page wood engraving "centerfold" in *Harper's Weekly* of January 28, 1860. His view of the frozen pond in the newly created Central Park, still raw and relatively treeless, is crowded with men and women together, enjoying the activity, showing off their pleasure and grace in the cold winter weather.

Some years later *Godey's* ran a three-page article, "Skating for Ladies," subtitled, "Why Ladies Ought to Skate, And Why They Do Not."[20] This article, written by a man, "J.L.M.," gives us a vivid sense of thoughts of the time concerning women's participation in outdoor activities. I quote it at length to show the attitudes women faced, the pervasiveness of those attitudes, and the distance women had to travel to overcome the limits of "women's sphere." Somewhat surprisingly, and probably unbeknownst to him, J.L.M.'s words also clearly defined issues of class and social expectations.

The writer allowed that he had skated since he was a schoolboy, but "personally speaking, I have always regretted that more ladies do not skate. . . . In cold Christmas weather, when a merry party was gathered in my father's house, it would have been so much pleasanter not to have had to leave the young ladies at home while we were at the pool." He admitted that once they arrived at "the pool," the men found "the lads from the village and not a few girls too." Meanwhile, back at home, what were the ladies doing? (Notice his inadvertent distinction between the outgoing, carefree "girls" of the village and the "young ladies" who stayed at home.) "They cannot ride; it would be cruel to the 'poor feet' of the horses, to say nothing of the danger of slippery roads." So they sat "around the fire and indulge in 'small talk'—I beg pardon—or they knit, crochet or embroider. . . . (I may remark *en passant*, that therein ladies have a great advantage, being able to make nimble and good use of their fingers while carrying on the most animated conversation, whereas the most gentlemen can, or, at least, the most they *do* do, under similar circumstances, is to smoke.)" So rather than sit, he urged them to try skating, as his sisters did, becoming his "happiest skating companions."

If the ladies did venture outside, it was to deliver sandwiches to the male skaters at the pool, pausing to watch them briefly (in a sharp enactment of my earlier observation that women just watched) before it became "painful, and they hurried back to the fireside for the remainder of the bright day." At best, they allowed themselves to be pushed around the ice on a converted "superannuated rocking-chair from the nursery." It was after such a day, the author added, that he undertook the task of teaching his sisters to skate, a skill much easier than most people believed, so long as they had confidence. He argued that skating is healthy, "as delightful an amusement as dancing," and one that women could do very well, just as gracefully. "If I can. . . induce ladies generally to follow the excellent example set by a few of their number," he wrote, "I am confident they will be thankful for the addition to their somewhat limited number of amusements, one of the purest and best sports practised by men."

All this notwithstanding, in his experience ladies did not skate, and he considered the reasons why. Here we are privy to a generation gap evident well over a hundred years ago. The author rails against an argument that would have teeth for the next three-quarters of a century:

> I shall first of all deal with the weakest objection raised against it; but it is one, though puerile and paltry, which I feel to be very general. Paterfamilias objects to his daughter's skating, because he thinks it is unfeminine. This is one of those deplorable notions with regard to 'proprieties'. . . . It is unfeminine for ladies to be healthy, good walkers, with an upright gait, and a frame that is physically able to endure as much watching and working, if need be, as they are willing to undergo? Nothing I know is more conducive to these qualities than skating. Yet, say how many fathers, it is "unladylike."

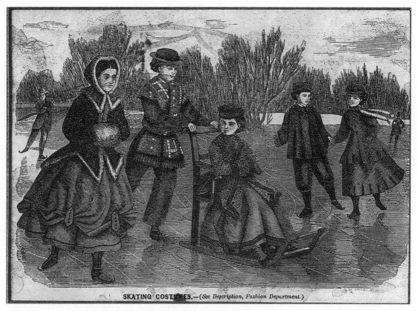

SKATING COSTUMES.—(*See Description, Fashion Department.*)

"Skating Costumes," 1869. Boys and girls enjoy the ice together. The one non-skater, perhaps a pre-learner, is pushed in a chair with runners. All are fashionably dressed, the girls in "short" skirts, modified to prevent tripping on their skates. Collection of the author.

Another difficulty he encountered was that of finding "a sufficiently private place for learning." Here we discover the circumstances under which a young woman might participate in any new sporting activity, not just skating. We shall see these conditions reiterated again and again over the years, whether with swimming and bathing, bicycling, or any other sport. The author insists that women must learn away from the eyes of strangers, and if under the tutelage of a man, it must be a brother or close friend: "It is, for obvious reasons, very desirable that a lady's first day on the ice should be only in the company of some few friends upon a pond not frequented by others. . . . A brother or a friend, used to the ice" might accompany her. "Another reason why skating is not general among women," he asserts. "is a natural objection each one feels towards taking the first step. That is, the first step among her own circle of friends. A few, a very few, ladies do skate, and have done so now for many years." His exhortation concludes, "It is a great folly, to say nothing of the positive wrong, to narrow the straitened limit of out-door amusements in which ladies are privileged to indulge."

His parting shot, a particularly American one, is to predict that the many ponds and rivers frozen during the wintertime, when "riding is generally impracticable," will create a greater attraction for skating, which will "be productive of more good than it ever has been in England."

Two months later, in *Godey's* February 1864 issue, "Rules For Skating" appeared under the heading "Hints About Health," taken from "Hall's Journal of Health." The seven hints range from avoiding strapping on the skate too tightly for fear of cutting off circulation ("a young lady at Boston lost a foot in this way") to wearing a veil over the face to prevent "fatal inflammation of the lungs." Skaters were not to sit down to rest "a single half minute" or stand still, or even to "stop a moment after the skates are taken off," to prevent becoming chilled. Walking home rather than riding was forbidden, since it would "almost certainly give a cold." And in light of the previous warnings, which make one wonder why anyone would ever want to skate at all, children and ladies were to limit their skating time to a mere hour. The seventh rule, though, really startles, if only because it makes us aware of the birth of another sport that did not take off until the next century: "The grace, exercise, and healthfulness of skating on the ice can be had, without any of its dangers, by the use of skates with rollers attached, on common floors; better, if covered with oil-cloth."[21] And, in case readers had missed it the first time around, *Godey's* repeated this last piece of advice in March, adding, "Little girls should learn skating this way; it is pleasant and safe exercise."[22]

Godey's seems to have been aware of the fashion trends, at least in certain circles, for that May it declared in its regular column "Letter From Paris" that "the thaw has put a stop to the pleasures of skating—and exercise which has been pursued by many of our leaders; the favorite lake in the Bois was the Suresne, because the Empress selected it, and was frequently seen upon it."[23] (This was the period of devotion to the empress Eugénie's fashion leadership, a period mourned at its passing by the *beau monde* because of the distressing vacuum it left in the fashion world.) Whatever the influences, skating became a regular pastime, one referred to several times in *Godey's* over the course of the next decade or more. As early as January 1868, just four years after the "J.L.M." article, the editor declared with nonchalance, "Until the last few years...[skating] was almost confined to [boys]; but now everybody skates, and ladies are especially renowned for their grace and agility."[24] By the 1870s, descriptions of skating costumes appeared along with those of other fashionable dresses as a matter of course.

If *Godey's* incorporated clothing for outdoor sporting activities into its standard reportage, it can be stated with unflinching authority that those outfits were attractive, meant to be seen, and bound firmly within current fashion standards. A short story in *Peterson's Magazine*, "The First Skating-Lesson," bears this out, and confirms that just as the clothing for croquet was chosen to attract, so was the clothing for skating. This story, written by a man, revolves around the pairing of a young couple at the end of a week-long Christmas party. It begins with the young woman's first attempt at skating, accompanied by the young man, of course. Tellingly, a complete description of their appearance virtually begins the tale:

> Amy Forsyth almost always looked pretty, but never prettier than she did standing there in her coquettish short dress, with its loosely-fitting velvet jacket, ermine-edged, a jaunty hat, with a floating feather, and her beautiful hair allowed to fall in loose, heavy waves about her shoulders. The rose-tints in her cheeks were deeper, and her eyes brighter than usual, from excitement and the fear which was not too strong to be pleasurable, enough to make her hold fast to Fred's two hands, so that he was inclined to think the nervousness was nicer than any Amazonian display of courage and skill.
>
> Fred, in his stunning winter array, made a very charming cavalier. He was only twenty-two, bright, witty, and highly cultivated—in every respect an agreeable companion.

The entire story, complete with all the flirtation, coyness, misunderstanding, and drama of the usual boy-meets-girl, boy-loses-girl, boy-gets-girl plot, revolves around skating and the dramatic possibilities it afforded (including crashing through the ice into the frigid water). Who could resist trying it out, especially when the romantic outcome was so inevitable?

Just as *Peterson's* reported the latest fads in its stories, *Godey's* kept up with the prevailing fashions from France. The orientation of the time was The Crinoline, synonymous with the Second Empire. Indeed, the label still sticks: the 1850s and 1860s are known to costume historians and others alike as the "Crinoline Era." François Boucher claims that at least part of the reason it stormed the fashion world was that, after the bourgeois reign of Louis-Philippe and the Revolution of 1848, women were "avid for luxury, for pleasure, and for *la toilette*," just as their grandmothers had been during the Empire Period. It was an era that "had money in abundance." It was a time to see and be seen at receptions, balls, spectacles, and fantasies; it called for experimentation and participation in new social pastimes of all sorts.[25] Sport was simply one of these.

Since both croquet and skating first appeared in the 1850s, the costumes naturally consisted of the wide, bell-shaped skirts supported by crinolines that characterized the era. This was also the triumph of *"la couture mécanique,"* as Boucher put it, consecrated by the Universal Exposition of 1855. Dressmakers, intoxicated by the speed of the sewing machine, had finally found relatively inexpensive ways to adorn the huge skirts, all in a reasonable amount of time. Out of their enthusiam came the excess that the Crinoline Era is famous for.[26] The designer Charles Frederick Worth, couturier to Eugénie, "Empress Crinoline," was an advocate of the fashion, and was abetted by the court painter extraordinaire, F. X. Winterhalter, who recorded it for posterity.

The crinoline itself was an underskirt made of horsehair and cotton or linen, starched and stiffened to support the wide skirts. As these broadened ever further, the additional weight of the yards of material led to the invention of the steel-banded cage, known as the cage crinoline. Although it seems hard to believe now because it made possible an ever-greater expanse of skirt, it was for its time a remarkable example of reform dress. Patented first in France in 1856, and easily manufactured by the new sewing machine, it eliminated the need for the heavy burden of multilayered crinolines proper, substituting instead a single steel-hooped petticoat.[27] In spite of this innovation, it took another two years for the skirt to reach its widest span, and two more years to refine the cage enough to respond to the movement of the body with a suppleness that hadn't existed in the earlier versions.[28] The timing was perfect for croquet and skating. Interestingly, although, according to *Godey's*, the empress skated on her "favorite lake in the Bois. . . the Suresne," the same article reveals that Eugénie *"never"* wore a cage. *Godey's* mused somewhat slyly that it was a

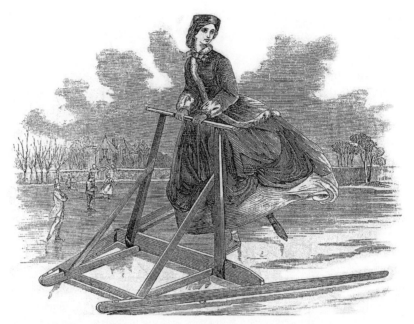

"Safety Skating Frame, for Beginners." Note the hoop shaping the shortened elevated overskirt. Despite the voluminous layering, the lower body seems to be vulnerable to winter's chill. *Godey's Lady's Book*, December 1863, 505.

"matter of curiosity to know how the Empress contrives always to appear with such well-setting skirts." Her "well-starched flounces," the writer sniffed, were "a costly contrivance, and. . .not suitable for those who take much walking exercise."[29] Or skating exercise either, it would appear, in spite of her alleged fondness for the Suresne.

Perhaps the reason why Eugénie shunned the cage in favor of the earlier and heavier versions of the crinoline had to do with the drawback that wearers and cartoonists alike dealt with. The cage had a tendency to dip and bob, to maintain a life of its own when circling a moving body. A good gust of wind could lift it high, even turn it inside out, much like an umbrella in a windstorm. Its bounce could not only dislodge "well-setting skirts" but also reveal all beneath. Thus feet, shoes and boots, legs and stockings, even pantalettes and petticoats became newly important articles of apparel and objects of erotic interest in the Crinoline Era. Women had been wearing drawers under their skirts for two or three decades by the 1850s, but the sudden and unplanned tilting of the covering skirts persuaded them to adopt

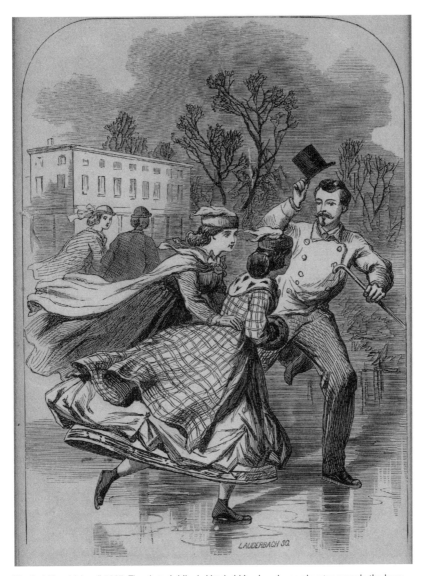

"On the Wissahickon," 1867. The skater's hiked skirt, held in place by an elevator, reveals the hoop underneath. Collection of the author.

pantalettes as a matter of course. And the more visible they were, the more decorative they became. Petticoats, too, lent themselves to a new and eye-catching display. Usually one petticoat would be worn over the cage to soften the line, and since it showed frequently, it became an object of exploitation (and here we begin to appreciate the scope of opportunities for lavish deco-ration that the sewing machine provided). It should come as no surprise that inveterate English walkers were the first to hitch up their skirts to allow eas-ier movement. It was Eugénie, though, who popularized the look after she saw it on a visit to England, took it home to France, and inspired the fashion world. By 1862, French fashion plates, those models for American copies, showed the newly hiked skirts. This in turn led to a wider use of mechani-cal devices to lift skirts (such as the "elevator" used by Winslow Homer's croquet players), first introduced in the late 1850s, but brought more into popular use in the 1860s. Mme. Demorest, the New Yorker whose emporium *Godey's* frequently touted, who published the *Mirror of Fashion* in 1862 and teamed with Ebenezer Butterick to publish the first paper sewing pat-terns in the United States, invented a "superior" device for the purpose.[30]

The English also led the way in the matter of stouter boots and stockings made in bright colors or stripes. Interestingly, the popularity of skating at this time not only led to a new awareness of smart boots for women, but in return, encouraged even more women to take up skating. Without the stur-dier shoes for women, the blades that strapped over them could never have held as well as they did or led ultimately to the skate still used today, with the blade attached directly to the boot sole.

Godey's, as usual, tells us all about the "new," yet cautions the reader in the telling. Here we see the interaction between the innovations for sport, certain accommodations for the weather, and the acceptable fashion of the period:

> The fashion for colored stockings has certainly extended since the skating mania. Naturally the ankles are visible during this exercise, and white stockings have a miserable effect with a colored petticoat. Never, therefore, have colored stockings appeared to such an advan-tage; plaid looked especially well. They are worn in silk, spun silk, and fine wool, and they are always selected to match the dress. The white silk stockings, which were abandoned last winter, are the only ones admitted during the present season for full evening dress.
>
> Boots are also made fantastically; with the present style of looping up the dresses, both in fine and wet weather, the feet are seen very

plainly. On fine days the dress is not drawn up so high as when the streets are muddy, but in all weathers the feet of pedestrians are, now-a-days, visible. Unless the precaution of drawing up the skirts was taken, considering their present length, even when made of the richest materials, they would not last more than a couple of days.[31]

That *Godey's* was something other than consistent is apparent in the "Fashions" article by Mrs. Hale in February 1864, just two months after J.L.M.'s plea to encourage skating among women. "Skating," declared *Godey's* rather surprisingly, "is now so universally recognized as an institution among ladies, as well as gentlemen, that not a little taste and ingenuity are exercised in getting up costumes, which will be at the same time warm, comfortable, convenient, and picturesque."[32] But what follows is a tribute to *Godey's* forward-looking, unfettered spirit, and a rare societal impress on the reform dress of the mid-century. For what Mrs. Hale goes on to describe is nothing less than the Turkish costume known by then as the bloomer, and the outfit that, modified, would become the standard exercise costume of the next couple of decades (a development discussed at length in Part Two).

"Most ladies," she writes, "content themselves with drawing up their soft woollen and merino dresses over gaily striped and ornamented underskirts." For the daring few, though, Mrs. Hale suggested that "the most suitable and admired of these [skating] costumes are made in French flannel, and consist of a Garibaldi, Turkish pants and a short skirt, which leaves the limbs free for exercise." Outfits she describes are elaborate, richly decorated, and made from expensive materials. "All these were made by Madame Demorest, although with patterns and a little ingenuity, they could be readily made at home." With this, Mrs. Hale was no doubt reminding her readers that patterns were available for order from Mme. Demorest, through both *Godey's* and, from 1862 on, Demorest's own magazine. It should be pointed out that the word "costume" was used exclusively here to label the reform Bloomer outfit, as in this passage:

The pants should be pretty wide, and drawn with an elastic band. Where it is not convenient to procure a costume, an ordinary walking dress, drawn up over a Balmoral skirt with one of Mme Demorest's excellent elevators, of which we gave our readers a description last

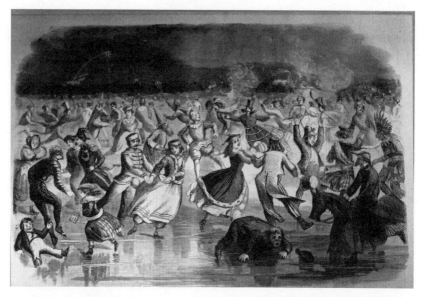

"Skating Carnival in Brooklyn, February 10, 1862." Note the woman of the central couple wearing bloomers under her skirt. Of all the people on the ice, she alone wears the "costume." *Harper's Weekly*, February 22, 1862, 125. Courtesy of Mount Holyoke College Special Collections and Archive.

month, answers just the same purpose. The only advantage of the regular costume is, that there is less weight to carry, and it is certainly more effective. A long skirt is, of course, worn over a skating dress in going to and from the place of rendezvous.[33]

This last sentence is surely the earliest admonition of its kind, but one that would appear over and over throughout the next several generations of clothing for sport and exercise. Indeed, the prohibition lasted well into the 1960s, when college women were expected to wear raincoats over their gym suits on the way to class.[34] As to "the only advantage of the regular costume," one would agree that weight reduction was a primary consideration, though perhaps additional warmth, particularly in the nether regions, would have run a close second. Still another, though again not acknowledged here, would be the ability to see one's feet clearly on the ice instead of having to peer over the hoopskirt, which would constantly be hiding the skates—and cracks and bumps in the ice—from view (not to mention the exposure should she fall). A final advantage might be to allow the skater to strap on her own skates when sitting down, since she would be able to see her own feet. Otherwise, someone else would have had to put her skates on for her.

As to the success of "the costume," it seems to have vanished without a trace, if indeed it was ever much worn at all. I have been able to find no other mention of pants for skating in any other source from that time on. We must wait until the 1930s to see them worn again for skating. From this earlier point on, then, clothing for skating, like clothing for croquet, was very much standard fashion fare, what "most ladies content themselves with." In fact, this suggests that women preferred to follow fashion rather than fly in the face of convention, no matter how sensible the innovation might be.

Skating and croquet, as we have seen, were both introduced at the same time, during the 1850s. Skating, a winter sport, required certain modifications in dress, if only to protect the wearer from the cold. By the 1860s, the skirt elevator was introduced to manipulate the huge crinolined skirts and was used not just for skating and croquet but for general purposes as well, such as rainy-day walking. Contemporary illustrations of skaters show that, when the outer skirt was lifted with such a device, the hooped petticoat underneath fell only to the mid-calf, leaving the lower calf, ankle, and foot clearly visible. Children's clothing for skating from the same decade shows outer skirts falling to the same length as the adults' underskirts. Such a length for women elsewhere was unthinkable at the time. *Godey's* did comment in 1867 that "short dresses, which have caused so much perturbation in the feminine world, have now become almost indispensable. They grow shorter and shorter; but do not be frightened, dear readers, we are not coming out as ballet dancers; though the upper skirt is short, the petticoat is of a suitable length."[35]

The shortened petticoat, used here to avoid the blades of skates, represented the first of decades of similar—and in most cases only—modification of clothing for sport. Safety in general must have been a factor, since it would have been impossible for the wearer of a cage to see her feet unless she bent far enough forward to allow the hoop to swing backwards. Surely this would have been, at the very least, an inconvenience, especially in the learning process. Indeed, it was for safety's sake (and not just on the ice) that the cage changed shape in the 1860s from bell to oval, flattening the skirt in front.

Skating, then, was a significant outdoor exercise, not only because it represents a beginning for women's participation in sports but also, like bathing and swimming, it was very much an inexpensive and democratic pastime. Unlike croquet, with its more aristocratic origins, skating was accessible to anybody who could afford a pair of blades to strap onto his or her boots and who had a frozen body of water nearby. In spite of the awkward and unavoidable clothing they wore for it, women took up skating by the thousands. Indeed, no matter how great the struggle, how restrictive the patriarch, how hampering the clothing, how difficult the journey, women wanted to leave the "warm fireside on a bright day," get outdoors, and, in the words of sports promotion in our own time, "just do it." And they did.

TAKING
UP
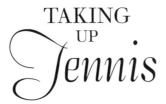
Tennis

THE FIRST REAL SPORT FOR WOMEN TO EMERGE FOLLOWING THE CRAZE FOR croquet was lawn tennis. Court tennis, or *jeu de paume*, as the French called it,
had been a sport of kings. Akin to handball, it was played on a walled court,
both indoors and out, from the misty depths of the medieval period. By the
sixteenth century, players used a rudimentary racquet instead of their bare
hands.[1] Henry VIII of England, who had a tennis court at Hampton Court,
was an accomplished player—"it is the prettiest thing in the world to see
him play," reported a foreign ambassador—and his inventories listed suits of
clothes designed specifically for tennis. Royal enthusiam dwindled considerably over time, and by the nineteenth century, tennis had become a game
played by rich Englishmen in their clubs. Needless to say, women were
excluded. By the 1870s, though, according to rumored sources, a Major Walter Clopton Wingfield (a source of the rumors himself, it is said), aware of
women's enthusiasm for croquet, suggested that tennis be moved exclusively
outdoors and that it include women. His motive wasn't altogether altruistic;
he apparently wanted to offer the men who partnered the women more of a
workout than croquet could provide. Accordingly, in London in 1869, he
invited friends to play his new game based on court tennis. It was not quite
the success he had hoped for, but after tweaking the rules, the size and shape
of the court, and the height of the net, four years later, in 1873, he once
again invited friends to play, this time in Nantclwyd, Wales. By December of

that year, he had patented his game under the name "Sphairistike." With the patent came an eight-page rule book, titled "Sphairistike or Lawn Tennis," with the subheading "The Major's Game of Lawn Tennis, Dedicated to the party assembled at Nantclwyd in December, 1873."[2]

However reminiscent of all other hand or racquet ball court games it was, and however many challenges arose to the story of its origins, it caught on. Within the next year, an American, Mary Ewing Outerbridge, watched British army officers play a version of the game while she was on vacation in Bermuda. She managed to buy a set of equipment and toted it home to New York, where she and her brother set up a court at the upper-class Staten Island Cricket and Baseball Club. Later that summer another American, William Appleton, established the game at a club in Nahant, Massachusetts. Almost immediately, then, tennis moved off private estates and became a club game. Back in England, the Marylebone Cricket Club took it on, as did the All England Croquet Club, which shrewdly added "Lawn Tennis" to its name. In fact, so popular was the upstart tennis that it shoved the staid—and aging—croquet aside. The All England dropped "Croquet" from their name and staged their first play-off at their club in Wimbledon in 1877. The rest, as they say, is history.[3] Almost simultaneously, tennis sprang up everywhere, usually under the auspices of the upper or upper-middle classes. By 1887 the *New York Tribune*, obviously in awe of the elite overtones of the game, reported:

> Tennis clubs have sprung up all over the country; playing continually improves; and numerous tournaments with valuable prizes are held each season. The elegant character of the game holds off the professionals; and lawn tennis continues the game of polite society, essentially one for ladies and gentlemen. The original game was the pastime of kings and nobles; and though the modern game is simple, fascinating and inexpensive, there still lingers about it the odor of aristocracy.
>
> During the past season 450 clubs have obtained courts at Prospect Park in Brooklyn.[4]

In spite of the claim of gentility, the very fact that some 450 clubs had appeared with such amazing speed in Brooklyn alone would suggest either that Brooklyn was a city of the gentry or that tennis didn't take long to democratize once it hit American shores. *Outing* magazine, whose very existence reflected the importance of the sports movement, also carried the banner of elitism. In 1881 it reassured ladies that tennis would never attract the lower orders, and that, should they wish to participate, they would be "in the company of persons in whose society [they are] accustomed to move."[5] And of course, even though it eventually welcomed the middle classes, tennis continues to enjoy an aura of social status.

Interestingly, the game of tennis as we know it today depended as much on two inventions as it did on any creator or upper-class enthusiasm. The first was the lawn mower, which coincided with the explosion of interest in croquet; the second was the invention of the rubber-core tennis ball. Although the cause and effect of the reel lawn mower strongly influenced the game of croquet, its impact was even greater on tennis, given the remarkable spread of the game. Indeed, at Wimbledon, at the All England Lawn Tennis Club, a sign over a lawn mower dating from around 1858 claims that without the invention of the mower, we would not be playing the game of lawn tennis we know today. The perfect green grass courts on which tennis was first played in the 1870s, and which gave the game its name, depended on the new machine.[6]

As for the ball, it represented a major difference between the earlier games of court tennis, or *jeu de paume*, and the game of lawn tennis, which needs a ball that bounces. Ancient balls were hard, made out of wool wrapped in leather strips. Because they had little or no bounce, they must have required a ferocious stroke to return off the floor or walls, which might explain how a man could even be killed by one, given enough misdirection. (Charles VIII of France is known to have been hit on the head and killed by such a solid, hard ball in 1498.)[7] In the eighteenth century, layers of strips of wool three-quarters of an inch wide, wrapped around a tight core of wool strips, were tied into place with a specific pattern of string, then covered with a white fabric and sewn in place, giving us the precursor of the fuzzy white tennis ball of recent times. What made the difference in the game, though, was the vulcanization of rubber, a process developed by the American Charles Goodyear in 1839. The India rubber that evolved from Goodyear's process was applied as a hollow lining for the new tennis ball, used from the beginnings of lawn tennis in the 1870s.[8]

Although men and women played tennis together from the time it was introduced in the 1870s, Wimbledon did not abandon the pattern of clubbish male exclusivity that had flourished for centuries until 1884. Actually, in view of the prevailing notions about women and their activities at that time, the 7-year lag seems remarkably short. Far from the grunts of exertion accompanying the strength and endurance that competitive tennis engenders today, tennis at that time required little running or hard exercise. In fact, players did little more than bat a ball back and forth across the net—"pat ball," as it was called. As for the clothing, the restrained and ladylike nature of the game was a blessing. Women in contemporary illustrations (and cartoons too, it might be added) are shown arrayed in up-to-the-minute fashion, which in the 1880s achieved the tightest fit of any decade of the century, or indeed any decade since. Not only were women stuffed into encasing sleeves, corsets, and bodices, but they were also bound by yards of draperies swathed around their knees and drawn up in the back to form the most protuberant bustle ever to confound fashion. Hats perched firmly in place, gloves covered the hands clutching the racquets (to say nothing of the trains of the gowns held in the other hand), and shoes as often as not had heels. Never mind: the women were not expected to actually run for the ball.

All the same, at least one reform dress for tennis appeared at the time. In their history of sports fashions, Phillis Cunnington and Alan Mansfield refer to a fashion illustration of a dark dress as tight as skin on a banana, torso outlined by a curvaceous corset, legs swathed in horizontal swags laced together in the front in a fetching criss-cross pattern and gathered into a bustle at the rear, with a skirt that fell in straight knife pleats to the ground. This dress, so it was claimed, was a splendid bow to the action of tennis. One might ask how. First, and most important, it was fashioned out of the new knitted wool cloth known as jersey. Because of the way jersey "gave," the tight sleeves would hold their shape but ease over the bent elbow or the reaching arm. Even the skirt, so fashionably slim over the entire lower body, was also designed to give. The lacing on the swag could be eased open, and the pleats at the bottom allowed the feet to move without excessive binding. So, clearly, at least some dressmakers had the interests of the players in mind when they set out to accommodate them.[9] It seems that in the early years of tennis's popularity, designers had to feel

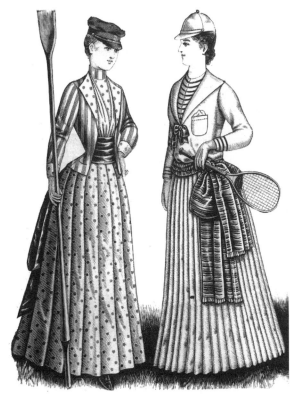

"Ladies' Outdoor and Indoor Garments" show the versatility of "outing costumes." Made from "striped, tinted and plain white flannels and tennis and outing cloths . . . appropriate for tennis, sea-side, mountain and general outdoor wear." The "ladies' yachting blouse and kilt skirt" on the right is accessorized with a tennis racquet. *The Delineator*, July 1889, 4.

their way into new styles. By 1890, they offered a somewhat generic "outing costume" that covered a number of needs. *The Delineator* advised its readers that "tennis suits, though originally designed for outing purposes, are frequently worn at the sea-shore or in the country until the evening. They are sufficiently *négligé* to produce perfect ease and comfort, and when prettily made, are dressy enough to be assumed with propriety during the afternoon." A Sterns Brothers catalogue from the summer of 1892 showed six "Ladies' Yachting and Tennis Costumes." Only one was designated specifically for tennis, and it seemed to bear no relationship to the game at all, except perhaps in its cost, which was decidedly elitist. The "navy or black serge" dress was designed with a tight, low-cut sleeveless bodice worn over a long-sleeved silk blouse with a high-necked collar adorned with a large bow. It cost $17.50. Perhaps the one accommodation to tennis appeared in a note below that offered a cotton cheviot blouse instead of the silk, at the reduced rate of $13.75.[10] But clearly the preferred ensemble was the one shown. The skirt, slim and flat-fronted with fullness at the back, fell to the toe tips, barely skimming the ground.[11]

It is therefore perhaps noteworthy that the second female winner at Wimbledon, the one who abandoned the "pat ball" game, was a mere fourteen years old at the time of her first victory there, in 1886. "Exuberant" is the word that comes to mind as we read descriptions of her. Her opponent, Miss Maud Watson, the reigning women's champion, complained that she "did not have the same chance of returning the ball as with the other ladies." The young Charlotte, or Lottie, Dod was a curiosity. Her close-cropped hair, "unusual height and strength," and "violent" strokes amazed spectators used to seeing a much more demure and temperate game. Should there be any doubt that only a certain class played tennis, Lottie's case seals it. She blithely dropped out of Wimbledon one year in the 1880s to take a cruise with a yachting party. But she returned the next year, won again, and kept at it, losing only four games in her entire career, retiring in 1893 at the ripe old age of twenty-one.[12]

One has to wonder if she would have been allowed to play with such vigor and effectiveness had she been an adult at the time of her first victory. Since technically she was still a child, it is very possible that a certain leniency may have been granted her in the matter of dress, allowing her skirts to be shorter, fuller, and more suitable for a girl of her age—and for freedom of movement. One photograph of her does exist, showing a young, pubescent, shapeless girl wearing a light-colored, loose-bodiced dress that obviously has no corset underneath, and is gathered into a widish, low-slung skirt draped over the hips, a style typical of the 1880s. Since the picture cuts her off somewhere around her knees, we can only guess at the length of her skirt. In overall effect, the dress is either "aesthetic" (that is, loose but body-conscious and unconfining, a look very much in tune with the 1880s) or childlike.[13] The sleeves are unusual for the decade: they are bracelet length and have a puffed cap, again suggestive of the aesthetic dress that foreshadowed the ballooning sleeves of the 1890s and very much looser than the formidably tight sleeves of the 1880s. The dress looks very

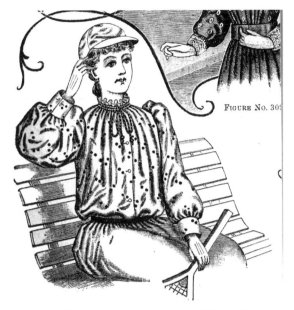

FIGURE No. 30

Tennis blouse, "spotted wash silk . . . particularly desirable for yachting, rowing and outdoor sports of all kinds." Note the tennis racquet held by her gloved hand. *The Delineator*, August 1891, 99

much like that of a young girl rather than a woman. Interestingly, a tennis blouse featured in *The Delineator* in August 1891 was fashioned on much the same lines. The tennis player is shown seated, clutching her racquet and fiddling with her hair, which is partly covered by a baseball-style cap (known as a "sports hat" at the time). Her sleeves are wide and gathered, with a high cap, and the neckline is high as well, and also gathered and ruffled. The waist or blouse (so-called because it blouses), is waist-length and very baggy, a most unusual style for the time.[14] To finish Lottie's outfit, in all likelihood her shoes would have been the new rubber-soled canvas tennis shoes, manufactured by the Spalding Company, a further development of the earlier "croquet sandal" that had appeared in the 1860s.[15] *The Delineator* details the range of popular styles in July 1892 (one year before Lottie Dod's retirement): "Tennis shoes are preferred low-cut and can be had in white canvas trimmed with white kid, and in russet and tan leather, the soles being always of rubber. Low shoes of black and tan ooze-leather [suede], with patent-leather tips, are also well liked for tennis. . . . The hosiery invariably matches the shoes."[16]

No one seems to have mentioned Lottie Dod's clothing at the time, so overwhelmed were they, one supposes, by her dynamic game. But perhaps after all, and certainly as she grew older, she dressed like the women she competed against. An insightful, even startling footnote to her story, especially for twenty-first-century readers, was recalled by a Major A. D. Mansfield, who saw her play a game of doubles in 1925 against two young women "wearing the modern type dress." According to Mansfield, Lottie, then in her fifties, managed to "[shake] up the girls" in the process. He concluded, "Here one can add that in the 1920s one still saw quite a number of the older women who still wore the pre-1914 kind of tennis dress and it was noticeable that some of them who were particularly small-waisted, and obviously tightly corseted, were particularly quick about the court."[17] A perfect gentleman, he named no names, leaving us wondering. But one thing Lottie Dod did do for the woman's game was to liven it up. Her successor, Blanche Bingley Hillyard, a woman with a powerful forehand, wore gloves for a better grip on the racquet, and often had a mass of bruises on her left shoulder from her own racquet's strong follow-through.[18] Such a thing would have been impossible had the game remained the gentle "pat ball" of the early 1880s.

As for the next teenager who conquered Wimbledon, the nature of her clothing is clearer. May Sutton was one of four tennis-playing sisters from Pasadena when she first came to Wimbledon in 1905 as a seventeen-year-old. That year she took the women's title, the first American ever to win the All England. Still teaching tennis back in California in 1972 at the age of eighty-two, she and her two older sisters, Violet and Florence, reminisced. (It must be remembered that this was the year before the famous Billie Jean King–Bobby Riggs match):

> "Girls were faster in our day," remembered Violet. . . . "We ran more. But it's a wonder we could move at all. Do you want to know what we wore? A long undershirt, pair of drawers, two petticoats, white linen corset cover, duck shirt, shirtwaist, long white silk stockings, and a floppy hat. We were soaking wet when we finished a match."
>
> "Girls today have a greater variety of strokes, but I believe we had more fight and speed, even though nobody ever dreamed of taking

lessons from a professional coach," said May. . . . "Girls played the net even then. It wasn't all baseline. Our weakest stroke was the serve. We just hit the ball up without much windup."

"But how May could hit that forehand!" enthused Florence. "She'd play all day without missing a forehand drive. She had power. When she won the nationals in 1904 and Wimbledon in 1905 and 1907, she weighed 160 pounds. Girls didn't worry about diets then. May even beat men. Our 'little sister' was the greatest of 'em all!"[19]

May Sutton may have been great, but she ran into some difficulties at Wimbledon because of her clothing. One of her competitors objected to the flash of ankle revealed by a shorter-than-customary skirt, and to her bare lower arm exposed by a daring short-sleeved blouse. After much crying foul by her opponent, she was allowed on center court only after she agreed to lengthen her skirt. Even though she was forced to comply with tradition, she is credited with leading the way to women's eventual emancipation from trailing skirts, high-necked shirts, and long sleeves.[20]

Violet mentioned a corset cover as one layer of apparel but said nothing of the corset itself. Because the girls were young at the time, they may not have worn corsets; or perhaps the "duck shirt" (called "health waists" in earlier times) that is mentioned—referring, one assumes, to a stiff cotton bodice made of the canvas-like fabric duck—was a substitute. But other women did wear them, even while playing championship tennis, as late as the 1920s. The U.S. women's amateur champion for 1910 (once again proving women's devotion to fashion rather than practicality) extolled their virtue, however vaguely, as "desirable for many reasons," not the least being that women looked better in them.[21]

Wimbledon has always been celebrated as a bastion of tradition and reverence for proper form. Scandalous clothing has been a concern since May Sutton's day. This has consisted of wearing any article of clothing that veers away from the traditional. Sutton's shortened skirt, probably no more than four to six inches from the ground, and her elbow-length sleeves were early examples. The knee-length, sleeveless Jean Patou dress that Suzanne Lenglen wore in 1919 was another; ankle socks, then shorts (for both men and, though short-lived, for women), colored rather than white clothing, and in the mid-1980s a form-fitting white nylon bodysuit were others. This last, worn by a player named Anne White, caused a great furor in 1985. The *Minneapolis Star and Tribune* reported, quoting umpire Alan Mills, in phrases eerily reminiscent of May Sutton's case:

> "The umpire [of the match] obviously decided she could wear it, but she was slightly fortunate to get away with it because it was not normal tennis attire . . . she won't be allowed to play in it again. She will be warned."
>
> The outfit brought photographers rushing to the court. Tennis fashion designer Teddy Tinling, who has chosen the garments of many top women players on the pro circuit, said: "She is quite within her rights. And she has a lovely figure to go with it."
>
> Wimbledon rules states [sic] that players must dress in predominantly white tennis clothing and that it must be appropriate.[22]

All these examples represent the continuous struggle for reform and change which doubtless will exist as long as Wimbledon itself does. In recent years, more color has finally come to the courts, and more skin is being revealed, as is evident in the high (and one could add questionable) design of Venus and Serena Williams's outfits. Nevertheless, the vestiges of Victorianism hold firm in that the women who play the strong, muscular, masculine, and brilliant tennis of today must still wear little dresses with skirts and underdrawers. The "public" face of sports which insisted that women wear skirts while playing remains with us, not only in this sport but in field hockey, too. *Plus ça change, plus ça reste.* And white remains the preferred color, making all others look, well, bad form. It has been suggested that tennis clothing is white because, when it started being worn at the turn of the century, it was not only a highly fashionable color for women's clothing, but also upper class. White clothes, hard to launder and keep pristine, were the prerogative of the rich. That alone, quite apart from the nature of the game itself, marked it as elite. Sparkling tennis whites are still the uniform of choice.

Wimbledon in the early days stood alone as the *ne plus ultra* of tennis. It still does. Even today, if a player is to accede anywhere to rules and regulations in the matter of dress, it will be there. But anyone who has picked up a racquet and headed off to the local courts knows very well that Wimbledon's regulation gear does not routinely appear on the folks playing on their neighborhood courts. As soon as the private clubs enter the picture, however, "appropriate" clothing becomes mandatory for their members. This is especially so in the matter of footwear, if only to protect the surface of the courts. Usually, though, it is the players themselves, who want to look as if they know something about the game, who dress accordingly and wear trim cotton polos or T-shirts with their primarily white skirts and shorts. But in the beginning, what did the average player wear? To gain some sense of that, we turn to Smith College, whose archives include early tennis photos.

Smith opened to educate women in 1875. Tennis appeared there just seven years later, two years before Wimbledon welcomed women's play. The first courts at Smith were simply wide grass lawns divided only by a net strung from two posts sunk into the ground. No lines divided up the court. We see these details in a remarkable stop-action photo from 1883. It shows four young ladies of the college dressed in dark, fashionably bustled and corseted dresses, smooth and slim at the skirt fronts, with long, tight—*very* tight—sleeves. One raises her arm to make her shot. The ball is clearly visible against the strings. But her hand is raised only shoulder high, in perfect form for a "pat ball" sort of game, and perfectly in keeping with the tight sleeve that sits very high in the armsceye.[23] The players' skirts fall to the instep; three women are bareheaded but one wears a hat. Another photograph from the same year shows three young ladies and a young man playing on the same grass. The man (a brother of one? a friend from Amherst College? an instructor?) is as fashionably and properly dressed as the girls, in a dark suit and a hat. By the following year, lines defining the boundaries of play had been laid out on the grass, but the clothes remained essentially the same. A studio portrait of a tennis foursome (perhaps the tennis team from Smith) dated 1884 verifies the high style that the women played in, complete to the corsets they wore. Even in the black and white photograph it is apparent that each girl wore a different color. Fashion plates from the 1880s offer a sportier alternative, often based on the yachting outfits of the time. One appeared in *Peterson's* in April 1888. Both fig-

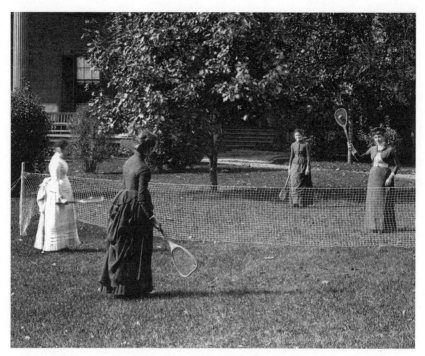

Tennis on the lawn at Smith College, 1883. Note the ball caught in midflight on the strings of the upraised racquet. Courtesy of Smith College Archives.

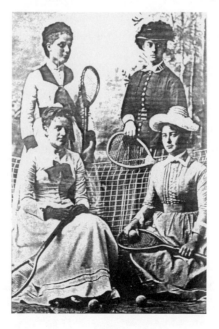

Smith College tennis team, 1884. All wear fashionable attire, tight enough to outline the corsets underneath. Courtesy of Smith College Archives.

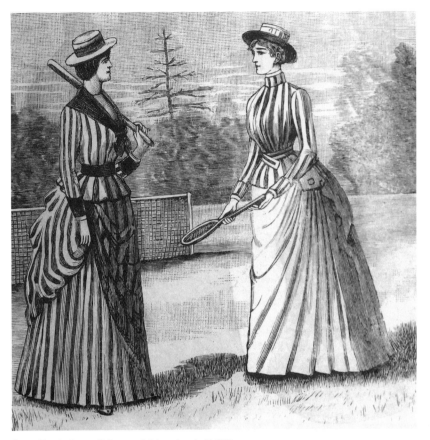

"Lawn-Tennis Gowns." *Peterson's Magazine*, April 1888.

ures keep the general 1880s silhouette with its tight jacket and bustled apron *tournure*, but they are boldly striped, echoing the blazers that men were wearing to play tennis at that time.[24] Both women wear very early versions—the earliest I have seen—of a man's boater on their heads.

Smith was not the only college to offer tennis. Bryn Mawr, opened in 1885, had tennis from the beginning. By 1892 it was a focus of athletic attention, and by the following year there was even a permanent court— one assumes indoors—for winter practice. That same year the college held an invitational tournament between the champions of Bryn Mawr and "the Harvard Annex" (later Radcliffe, now Harvard), as well as three students from Girton College, Oxford, who happened to be studying at Bryn

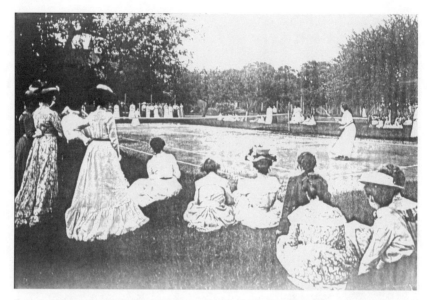

Smith College tennis tournament, 1901. Shorter skirts and rolled sleeves on the players contrast with the trained dresses of the spectators. Courtesy of Smith College Archives

Mawr. Miss Whittelsey of the Annex won the day.[25] No doubt they all wore mixed colors in their game. White became fashionable for tennis only after the turn of the century, when it became fashionable for women's clothing in general. An ad in *The Delineator* in August 1894 offered a "Manual of Lawn Tennis" (which was written, incidently, by that same Miss Whittelsey from Harvard Annex, who was referred to in the ad as "a well-known authority"). It shows a highly decorative leg-o'-mutton-sleeved outing dress, dark in color, with matching waist and four-gored skirt, trimmed lavishly with zig-zag braid at the hem and revers of the bodice. It is worn with a broad-brimmed, wired bow-trimmed hat and dark gloves. The ad also shows a voluminous-sleeved shirtwaist blouse worn with a dark full skirt.[26] In 1895, photographs show skirts and waists (or blouses) being worn in the style of the "tailor-made"—that is, menswear adapted for women—but again in more than one color. Here too the skirts are full-length. Only in a 1901 Smith photograph are we able to spot a difference in the clothing: by this time the players wear white, roll their sleeves to the elbow, and sport skirts short enough to show their feet. When we compare the players in this picture with the spectators, who are fashionably dressed with pompadour hairdos, many with elaborate hats, and even wearing dresses with trains, we understand that finally we are seeing what may be called a specifically designed tennis costume.

Here at Smith, then, this new modified outfit had evolved a full four years before May Sutton was chastised for wearing essentially the same sort of thing at Wimbledon. Probably it had appeared elsewhere as well, at the many colleges that offered tennis for their students. By 1909 this modified dress for sport was the preferred tournament wear, even in England. That year, Mrs. Sterry, British ladies' champion for the fifth time in a row, confided, "To my mind nothing looks smarter or more in keeping with the game than a nice clinging white skirt (about two inches off the ground), white blouse, white band, and a pale coloured silk tie and white collar." Her photo, in Elizabeth Ewing's *History of Twentieth-Century Fashion*, shows a white man's style shirtwaist with standard shirt sleeves, French cuffs with gold links, a high, stiff collar (we can't see the tie), a white skirt that looks like linen, smoothly gored to flare gracefully at her ankles, a firm and tight wide belt, and black stockings and shoes.[27] Like the players today, she wears earrings. So the special tennis dress was on its way by the first decade of the twentieth century, clearly modified from the fashion wear, the "tailor-mades," of the New Woman of the day, in response to the demands of sport.

Change came slowly to tennis, tied as it was to the authority and tradition of a powerful governing organization such as the English Lawn Tennis Association—or, in America, the United States Lawn Tennis Association. Since it was men who made the rules of the game, men enforced the rules and the fashion of play. In Part Two, we will see how gym clothing, formulated on the women's college campuses of the United States, had changed the rules of dress by the last quarter of the nineteenth century, introducing new concepts of comfort, practicality, and freedom of movement. College girls borrowed ideas from their brothers, stealing their turtlenecks and cardigans to accompany the baggy bloomers or significantly shorter skirts they wore to play outdoor sports. But such sensible clothing was never allowed for public wear by the male establishment. The short skirt came to

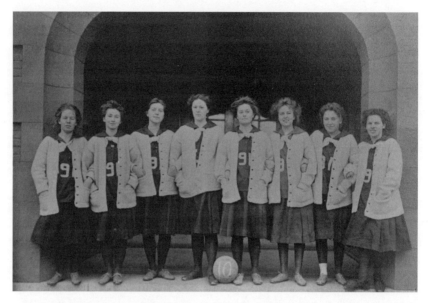

Mount Holyoke College basketball team in their outdoor uniform, 1910. Their knee-length skirts predated fashion by a decade. Courtesy of Mount Holyoke College Special Collections and Archive.

tennis only at the beginning of the 1920s, and sweaters were introduced, as accessories only, in the same period. But the knee-length skirt had been introduced for campus sports wear as early as 1910, and worn at international gymnastic events as early as 1912. Thus, the "shockingly" innovative short tennis dress designed by Patou for Suzanne Lenglen in 1919 was in reality a full ten years behind its prototype. Clearly, however, it was a style whose time had come. Lenglen's appearance at Wimbledon is described by Lord Aberdare in his *Story of Tennis*:

> Suzanne acquired strength and pace of shot by playing with men, and
> for playing a man's type of game she needed freedom of movement.
> Off came the suspender belt, and she supported her stockings by means
> of garters above the knee; off came the petticoat and she wore only a
> short pleated skirt; off came the long sleeves and she wore a neat short-
> sleeved vest. Her first appearance at Wimbledon caused much com-
> ment, but the success of her outfit led to its adoption by others. In her
> first championship, she wore a white hat but on subsequent occasions

she wore a brightly colored bandeau which was outstandingly popular until challenged by Miss Helen Wills's eyeshade in 1924.[28]

The straight line of her outfit echoed the bloomer-middy gym suit combination that had been introduced over a decade before, and confirmed the no-waist waistline that grew out of the high-waisted look of the 1910s. This was the combination of no waist, short sleeves, and knee-length skirt that soon captured the world. Even so, skirts remained longer for a few more years, but finally they too crept up to match Lenglen's Patou dress. In fact, Lenglen's entire look became the rage of the twenties: her bandeau— or "headache band," as it became known—was copied everywhere, as were her "rolled" stockings, which, teamed with knee-length pleated skirts, became the symbol of the flapper. For the first time, then, we see a sports figure influencing fashion in a complete, recognizable, and instantaneous way. The media had done their part; magazines and newsreels broadcast Lenglen's image all over the world. But the look had already appeared ten years earlier, in the women's colleges.

Other innovations at Wimbledon and Forest Hills in the 1930s, such as Mrs. Fearnley Whittingstall's short socks in 1931, had been accepted as normal gym wear for some time before they were paraded in the very visible public forum of international tennis. For example, the *Boston Herald* had published a photograph, "Girls Who Started in First Women's Intercollegiate Tournament," on June 25, 1929. The girls wear one-piece dresses, cut just to or at the knee, either with cap sleeves or completely sleeveless. Several wear headache bands. Anklets and white tennis shoes complete the outfits, even though some of the girls wear their anklets over long stockings, rolled above the knee (two years before Mrs. Whittingstall's socks debuted at Wimbledon). Alice Marble's much-talked-about shorts, worn first in 1933, broke a barrier, and even though by the end of the 1930s men routinely wore them at Wimbledon, shorts for women never really did catch on in tennis circles. Ironically, shorts are worn everywhere else for hot weather leisure wear—but not at Wimbledon. Women still wear little skirts for serious tennis. Perhaps from this we can conclude that the form of the new outfit came about first in the privacy of the campus testing ground, but it took the fashion-conscious stamp of approval that fame and international press coverage could bring in order to deliver the critically important message of acceptability to the world of women's fashion. Both had to be present. By the mid-thirties, then, in the years immediately prior to World War II, we see the merging of the two separate streams, the "private" gym costume and the "public" sports dress, into a new and fashionable kind of clothing, easy, sensible, and with interchangeable parts, that within another decade or two would start on the path of conquering the world.

BATHING
AND
$\mathcal{S}wimming$

Seeking a "Sensible Costume"

THE OUTDOOR LAWN GAMES OF CROQUET AND TENNIS NUDGED WOMEN INTO a new awareness of the need for more suitable clothing for sport. In spite of this, sporting dress for both activities remained firmly within the boundaries of the conventional. Other kinds of leisure activity enjoyed at the same time, however, forced thinking—and clothing—in new directions. Even more influential in bringing about change was the popularity of swimming and bathing. And the clothing for bathing had much further to go. James Laver, the keen-eyed and witty observer of clothing and its role in society, once wrote that "the only sensible costume for bathing in is no costume at all."[1] However much one might agree with him, rigid standards of modesty and the mid-nineteenth-century introduction of mixed bathing got in the way. The trouble was that when the body got wet, no matter how voluminous the drapery around it, it had a tendency to reveal itself under the sodden and clinging layers that were meant to hide it. Thus for decades the goal was to offer unfailing coverage, thereby retaining appropriate modesty while also allowing necessary freedom of movement. Clearly, this was not an easy assignment.[2]

The history of bathing and swimming dress reflects that uneasiness, that ambivalence. Until the middle of the nineteenth century, swimming had largely been the activity of men, while bathing—that is, dipping into the water, often in the name of healthful duty—was regarded as quite a different pastime, often a feminine one. The water cures of earlier decades had generated spas, which very properly kept the sexes apart even as they probably increased sexual interest by the very act of doing so. (We have seen how gleefully both men and women came together to play croquet.) The spa's water activities inevitably led women to seek the greater freedom of bathing in the ocean and lakes. Early on this too was controlled. Seaside resorts used red and white flags to carefully designate and limit the times when men and women could swim. Often each sex had its own separate section of the beach until, again inevitably, they recognized the pleasures of joining together in mixed bathing. People quickly realized that this activity too—just like croquet—encouraged flirting and courting.[3] Americans embraced this notion much earlier than their English counterparts. In an age of dubious acceptance of exercise in any form and rigorous adherence to role behavior, climate must have played a critical part. Relief from summer heat is rarely a factor in England. In 1833 a British visitor to the United States commented on the mixed bathing he saw, but added that since the parties always went into the water fully dressed, he could see no great violation of modesty. In any event, "even though they were completely clothed, few females dared to go into water where one had to be accompanied by a man."[4] In spite of these restrictions, by 1846 mixed bathing had become "the fashion all along the Atlantic coast."[5]

Until that time, men frequently bathed or swam nude, while women covered themselves in long, loose, and flowing dresses of a canvas-like material. Essentially heavy chemises or tent-like cloaks, when wet these ballooned out from the body, allowing freedom of movement for the arms and legs. Women entered the water from the privacy of small "bathing machines," which were little changing huts on wheels that could be pulled down to the edge of the water. Often brawny female attendants were on hand to help them paddle away from the steps of the changing houses, supporting them as they went through the motions of "swimming" and keeping them safely away from prying eyes. Swimming per se came very slowly to women, possibly because, until the second decade of the twentieth century, the clothing they had to wear would have pulled them to the bottom like a stone. Even after the reform in bathing suits, American women remained timid swimmers. Nevertheless, as early as September 1873 *Godey's* described a "swimming belt of bootstrapping ornamented with embroidery . . . used by children and grown-up people in learning to swim."[6] This sounds like some

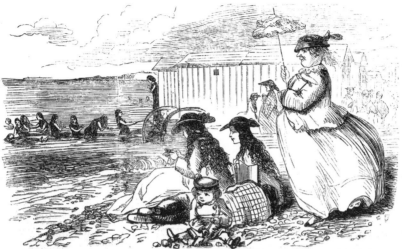

"THE WORST OF WEARING ONE'S BACK HAIR DOWN IS THAT IT MAKES THE YOUNG MEN STARE SO!"

"The worst of wearing one's back hair down is that it makes the young men stare so!" Segregated bathing, complete with changing houses or "bathing machines" that were rolled to the edge of the water. *Harper's Weekly*, September 18, 1858. Courtesy of Mount Holyoke College Special Collections and Archive.

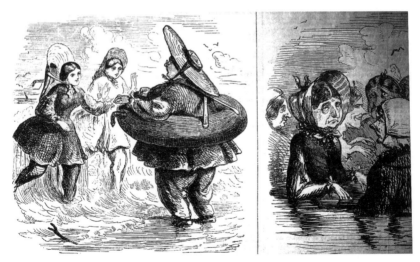

"Oh! Aunty dear, do come and duck under the wave. You've no idea how delicious it is!" Simple covered dresses of the 1850s, cut off above the knee, worn with straight-legged but loose trousers, in the bloomer style. *Harper's Weekly*, September 4, 1858. Courtesy of Mount Holyoke College Special Collections and Archive.

sort of harness for the attendant to clutch, and it sounds heavy besides. But from this we may assume that at least a small number of women were actually learning to swim rather than just paddling or playing in the water.

Swimming pools were being built throughout the country during these years, and colleges, even women's colleges, followed the trend. Goucher had one of the first, in 1888. By 1916, more than 32,000 women (out of a total U.S. population of 101,961,000, slightly fewer than half of whom were women) entered swimming programs offered by the YWCA. Clearly, the swimming population was not large; but it would seem that those who did swim were enthusiastic, because the following year the Women's Swimming Association of New York was officially organized to promote national and international competition for women.[7] In the next chapter I look more closely at this group and its success three years later at the 1920 Olympic Games. But first it is important to realize what went before, and how far those women had to come to achieve their international triumph.

According to the argument I have presented so far, we should find that the clothing for water activities in these years was fashion-oriented because it was worn when men and women interacted together out-of-doors. Such simplicity when speaking of swimming and bathing is merely a fond hope. The reality is much more complicated. The requirements of clothing for going into the water are unlike any other, and called for a very different development from all the other sporting wear discussed in this book. Certainly male influence played its part, pushing the early separation of bathing dress into a fashion-conscious mode while functional dress for swimming struggled for existence as late as the 1920s. The ambivalence I noted earlier is clear as we look at the clothes.

Obviously, the clothing for bathing and swimming is unique in that its function is to protect the body while allowing movement in the water. When wet, it becomes heavy and therefore sharply counterproductive to the purpose for which it is designed. Even worse, wet fabric often becomes translucent or even transparent. It clings to the surface underneath and reveals the form supporting it. In an age of militant modesty, these characteristics could and did present embarrassing problems for bathers. The solution in the late 1850s was to cover the body in several layers of loosely fitting but sturdy clothing, modeled on the bloomer costume of the time.

This outfit became the prototype for all women's bathing suits for the next half century.[8] Briefly, it consisted of a baggy, blouse-topped dress, "short" for its time, cut to the mid-calf and worn with a belt to gather in the fullness. With it, a pair of matching Turkish trousers was gathered at the ankle and finished with a ruffle. Often a short cape or "talma" was included to throw over the shoulders after emerging from the dip.[9] The cape's purpose was twofold: it would provide warmth if needed and, of equal importance, a modest covering should the "figure" suddenly be revealed too prominently. In other words, the outfit was cut similarly to the housedresses of the period, but modified with a shorter and narrower skirt to be worn over a pair of trousers rather than the customary petticoat. In this it was exactly like the reform bloomer or the exercise suit. Though modified over the next decades, it basically stayed within those boundaries.

Even—or perhaps especially—fashion magazines had grave difficulties in finding complimentary things to say about such costumes. In 1854 *Frank Leslie's Ladies Gazette of Fashion* started out encouragingly, but gave up in frustration, blurted out the truth, then turned finally to a straightforward description:

> [No. 7] is one of those bathing dresses so necessary to a seaside excursion or residence. If the invigorating sea-bath is to be enjoyed as it should be. The material is common Scotch plaid, green and red, in alternate checks. It is cut short in the bloomer fashion, which though very convenient when half veiled in snowy surf ought to astonish the sharks themselves on dry land. But a bathing dress is only intended for convenience, and the least idea of making it elegant would be preposterous. The dress is made with a loose skirt set into an old-fashioned tight yoke and gathered around the waist with a plaid belt; it is cut short, leaving the feet and ankles free. Long bishop-sleeves fastened around the wrist with a band protect the arm. The pantalettes are made loose and fastened around the ankles with narrow bands.[10]

Peterson's Magazine had to agree two years later that it was not a great-looking outfit, though at least *Peterson's* thought that with a little embellishing it might possibly be improved: "Bathing-dresses, although generally

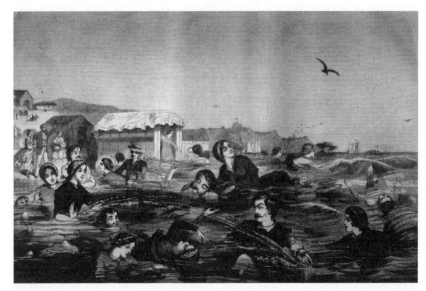

"The Bathe at Newport." Winslow Homer caught the delights of mixed bathing even as he recorded the encompassing clothing for the activity. *Harper's Weekly*, September 4, 1858. Courtesy of Mount Holyoke College Special Collections and Archive.

very unbecoming can be made to look very prettily with a little taste. If the dress is of a plain color, such as grey, blue or brown, a trimming of the talma, collar, yoke, ruffles, etc. . . . . of crimson, green or scarlet, is a great addition."[11] That it was discussed in the *Gazette of Fashion* and *Peterson's* at all is in some measure an indication that women were beginning to need such a costume. And of course, the dress was just the beginning. To complete the outfit, the wearer needed an oil cap to protect her hair from the water, a straw hat and lisle gloves to protect her face and hands from the sun, and gum shoes to protect her feet from whatever lurked on the bottom. One can only marvel at women's determination to partake in the activity at all when the entire body was swathed so completely.

Historians and fashion magazines notwithstanding, Winslow Homer recorded the bathing scene at the popular seaside resort at Newport for *Harper's Weekly* in 1858. He gives us a different picture from the ones we have seen so far. There is no doubt that the separation of the sexes was maintained with all the devices known to man, but how effective they were is another matter. Human nature has a tendency to find its own level. Such seems to be the case here. Men and women in Homer's scene gambol together in the waves, a few men supporting women to help them "swim." An occasional bare female foot and calf kicking into the air show below the billowing skirts. At least one woman's sleeves reach only to her elbow. Many women wear caps on their heads, but none in the water wears a straw bonnet, although several watching from the beach do. Claudia Kidwell has argued that Homer fell victim to youthful artistic license in depicting these swimmers so, and she may be right. A counterargument can be made, however, that although fashion magazines have always dictated a certain mode of dress, complete in every detail, many women stubbornly refuse to follow a slavish interpretation of the rules. And, given the "summer girl at the seashore" nature of the activity and the forward-thinking type of woman partaking of it in the 1850s, it seems quite probable that Homer did indeed record what he saw. He certainly had a precise eye for detail, in clothing and everything else, as his croquet prints, paintings, and other works attest. I would argue that his is likely a truer representation of the clothing worn at the time than the fashion prints, formalized as they were. In that era before rotogravure, artists like Homer were hired to record, not reinterpret.

The ladies' magazines kept their eye on developments in bathing costumes. They supported the Turkish trouser or pantaloon suit, but sometimes even they despaired, particularly when it came to fabrics. In 1864 *Godey's* sighed,

There is no dress so easy of accomplishment as a neat, tasteful and comfortable bathing dress; and yet, sometimes, when watching bathers at the sea-side, one is tempted to believe such an achievement impossible.

Instead of the usual flannel, Mme. Demorest is making bathing dresses of moreen, and considers this material better adapted to the purpose. It is of a strong, firm texture; not too heavy, does not cling to the person after being in the water, as it immediately drains off.[12]

This article not only illustrated these suits but instructed about decoration and construction. The suits "should of course be lined, except the skirt," in, the editors suggested, a very thin muslin with "just sufficient texture to make it smooth." They even proposed that some enterprising fashion leader at Newport or Cape May add a havelock (a cloth extension that would cover the back of the neck) to a lady's bathing hat, for "it is so disagreeable to have the sun beating down on one's neck, which it will do, in spite of the wide-brimmed hats."[13]

Englishwomen tended to be more relaxed in their swimming dress than Americans. They found it perfectly acceptable, for example, to wear a suit of pantaloons and bloused top, skirtless, while Americans clung to the more modest additional layer of a skirt. One reason was that as a rule, Englishwomen actually swam more than American women. American women who did adopt the English style were regarded as "masculine" and "fast," though by 1869 the costume was grudgingly permitted for "expert swimmers who do not wish to be encumbered with bulky clothing."[14] Probably this greater freedom in dress also had to do with the English segregation of men and women at the seaside until the end of the century. Women might well reason that since men could not see them anyway, they would not need to cover their pant legs with a skirt. This too is most likely why Englishwomen early on abandoned the long black stockings that Americans wore well into the twentieth century to complete their bathing outfits—a distinguishing characteristic in telling English images from American.

This bare-legged look in the fashion plates can be confusing. American publications showed illustrations of young women at the shore with their skirted suits and bare legs throughout the last decades of the nineteenth century. But magazines of the period were notorious for "borrowing" (sometimes over and over again, for many years) the fashion plates, or indeed any illustrations, from any source they could lay their hands on.[15] Thus European publications provided many images, however illegally copied, both for one another and for the American press. Many of the styles that were fashionable abroad were not necessarily either in fashion or acceptable in the more puritanical United States. Genuinely American sources—Charles Dana Gibson comes to mind—invariably clothed bathers from head (or, latterly, neck) to toe, always including those ubiquitous long black stockings as an inevitable part of the ensemble.

It is easy to see that bathing costumes, in their outer layers at least, by this time followed the dictates of fashion even though they included shortened skirts and the trousers that were prohibited for women anywhere else but in

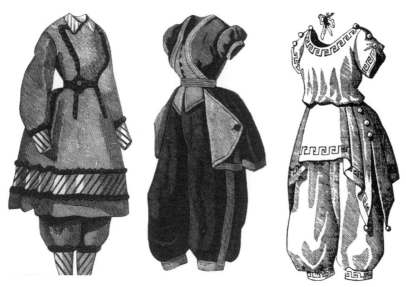

Left and center: Bathing dresses. These two outfits have moved beyond the unfashionable bloomer costume of the 1850s and 1860s to incorporate dressmaker details of the 1870s, including the suggestion of corsetry and bustles, even as they keep the trousers that scandalized the generation before. *Peterson's Magazine,* July 1870. *Right:* Bathing dress. Echoing the fad for classical motifs enjoying a revival, this outfit is daring for its time, with cap sleeves and a blouse top that barely covers the baggy pants below. *Peterson's Magazine,* July 1870.

sex-segregated exercise. In 1870 *Peterson's* showed that year's version of the bloomer as bathing dress, made out of black serge (a woollen material), fully covering with long sleeves, matching wool "leglets" that stopped at the ankle, and a leather belt. Even a bustle is suggested in the line of the back.[16] Along with this, however, were two other, rather more daring bathing dresses, both with short sleeves and draperies instead of complete skirts. One, made out of white flannel, was Greek-inspired, with a Greek key border around the tunic's scooped neckline and at the cuffs of both the sleeves and the baggy knee-length pants. The other, in black merino (also wool), has an almost military look, with a blue cashmere stripe down the side seam of the baggy mid-calf trousers and the half-skirt buttoned back at the hip, revealing a matching blue cashmere facing.[17] Rarely does one see so much attention to the trousers in the United States at this time; usually they were carefully covered by a skirt. These styles were obviously more English in tone than American; probably the plates were taken directly from European sources.

In July of the following year, 1871, *Godey's* introduced a new swimming outfit. An article titled "Ladies' Bathing Dresses" declared: "Great reforms have been made within the past few years in the bathing dresses worn by ladies." And "great reform was needed," they added, "for the preservation of modesty as well as of health and comfort." Swimming in the old long, loose gown, "apt to dab wet and flabby against the bather as she left the water," the writer recalled, "was very nearly something miraculous. Even in dipping in and out of the water, it would cling around the legs and impede freedom of motion. The very greatest objection of all was, that occasionally the air filled it, or the wind caught it, as the bather rose above the surface of the waves, and bore it up above the crest of the water like a balloon."[18]

The new outfit, appearing, it would seem, none too soon, was French in origin. In its description we can see the new thinking—and, it would follow, greater acceptance—not just for specially designed, lighter bathing clothing but for bathing itself. Its trim design prevented the embarrassment caused by the old dress. It had a short blouse, with or without sleeves, another innovation that had been introduced, as we have seen, the year before, and it was worn belted. The "trowsers" were to be no fuller than was "absolutely necessary, for the less material used the better; the more there is employed, the heavier the gown will be when saturated with water. . . . A costume will take about five yards." Colored flannel—undoubtedly wool—was recommended, but serge, of dark blue or brown, was even better. Fabrics of wool and cotton mixed puckered in water, so were unsuitable, and linen (specifically brown Holland) was not suitable either. Wool, obviously, was preferred. So was the natural, corsetless body, *Godey's* declared, for the sake of health and beauty.[19]

The 1880s suit, essentially similar to the earlier ones but pared down even further, kept the general line of 1880s fashion wear, which tended to be leaner and narrower. By this time the suit had modified to combine the bodice and trousers into a neat one-piece garment, very much like the English one but with the American addition of a separate skirt, falling just below the knee to conceal "the figure." Combination underwear had been introduced in the previous decade, and this, in addition to the English version, may have had its influence. The short sleeves, introduced at the beginning of the 1870s, came into their own in the 1890s, when short puffed sleeves were the height of fashion. The trousers, now knee-length bloomers

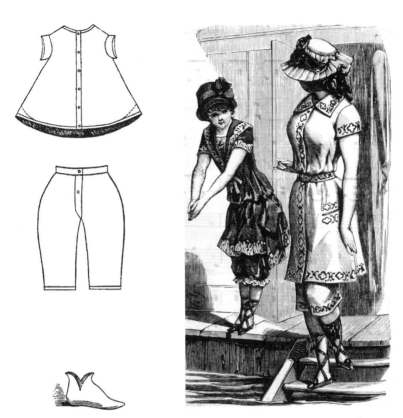

Left: New, reformed, French-style bathing dress: simpler, cleaner, shorter in top, trousers, and sleeves. *Godey's Lady's Book,* July 1871, 43. *Right:* "New Style Bathing Dresses." The child's (on the left) is bloused below the waist in the fashion of children's dress in the 1880s. It has a hint of bustle gathered at the back, but foreshadows the sailor collar that will characterize women's bathing dresses for over a quarter of a century. Note the sleeves and the trousers on both have shortened. *Peterson's Magazine,* August 1882, 68.

or knickerbockers the same length as the overskirt, used the new elastic to gather the fabric at the knee and waist. Sailor collars, decorative stripes, and nautical designs gave a jaunty, sportive look for the first time. Gone were the dressmaker details of earlier styles; instead a new, sleeker type of dress specifically for sport had taken their place. By now, a woman had the choice of wearing the overskirt or leaving it off while in the water if she really wanted to swim rather than paddle. Hats of oiled silk or waxed linen, often with wire to hold the brims stiff, held the masses of piled-high hair in check, and bathing sandals, oxfords, or slippers protected the feet. Except for these and the overskirt usually worn in the United States, the outfit

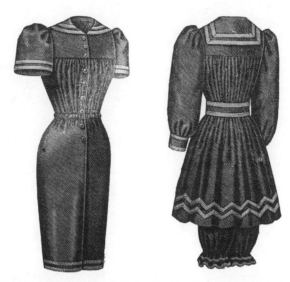

Peterson's offered readers options in their choice of bathing dresses. Here, the basic design with or without a skirt, long sleeves, or gathered pants. *Peterson's Magazine*, 1890s.

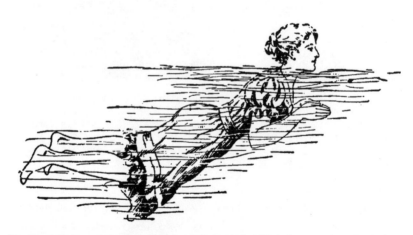

"The Breast Stroke . . . being the easiest, is usually taught first." Not all women chose the sleeker, skirtless swimming dress. *Peterson's Magazine*, August 1895, 222.

looked just like the gymnastic suit that had emerged at the same time. In fact, patterns of the entire period, from as early as the 1860s advertised the same suit as either a gym suit or a bathing costume.

In June 1896 *Harper's Bazar* pointed out how far bathing dress had come, but in the telling indirectly suggested that an acceptable solution had finally been attained and no further innovation was needed. The dresses "vary very little from year to year," the writer remarked; describing the old costume in order to demonstrate how modern and exceptionally fine the new one was:

> There will be no danger of a change in fashion before [the summer months] . . . since the great change from the so-considered modest costume of the most hideous gray flannel which used to be considered the correct thing. These were made, it will be remembered, with long full trousers reaching to the ankle and finished with a frill, and a full blouse to which was attached an exceedingly scanty skirt. The sleeves were made to the wrist, and a big straw hat completely hid all identity of the wearer. The present style of bathing dress, which has been in fashion for the last few years, is a very full skirt which reaches just far enough below the knee to cover the full knickerbockers or tights which are worn. The upper part of the costume consists of a blouse waist, sometimes made with a deep yoke back and front, and three box-pleats from yoke to belt; a high turn-over collar under which is worn a bright silk neck-tie is the finish, and the big puffed sleeves reach half-way down the arm. Such a dress as this, made of black serge or mohair, is considered the most correct model; but there are a great many dresses made with the sailor blouse instead, and broad sailor collar of some bright material, like turkey red.

The magazine justified its preference for serge and mohair (both firm wools) as being "wiry materials [that] shed the water more quickly than does the flannel." It assured readers that the only acceptable sleeves were the "big puffs," which allowed "full play to the arms while swimming," and that "well-fitting stockings are a very important part of the costume." Prospective swimmers were advised to buy them a size smaller than usual so they would not stretch out too much and get baggy when wet. High necks prevented "burning by the sun." The final piece of advice concerned corsets. Here, we become aware of the power of the women's magazines. In spite of the earlier admonition to abandon corsets while bathing, *Harper's Bazar* left little room for discussion: "Unless a woman is very slender, bathing

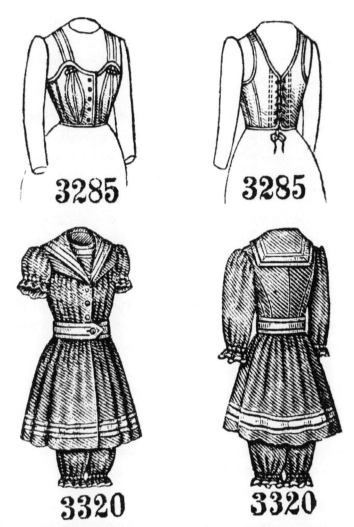

Pattern for a bathing corset: "a want that has long been experienced by fastidious bathers." Lighter in weight and boning, the corset was believed to be a necessity under outfits for swimming. *The Delineator*, July 1890, 65.

corsets should be worn. If they are not laced tightly they are a help instead of a hindrance in swimming, and some support is needed for a figure that is accustomed to wearing stays."[20]

It is important to remember at this juncture that corsets were as much a part of women's dress in the nineteenth century as brassieres are today. And anyone who might be tempted to gasp and giggle at the notion of wearing a corset while swimming should perhaps be reminded that twenty-first-century swimwear is often a marvel of both the pattern maker's and the engineer's art. Even today, when high-fashion swimwear is minimal and revealing in ways never before even imagined, much of it is still designed to support, mold, hold, and hide "unless a woman is very slender." Technology has advanced to the point where elastic fibers built in to the fabric of the suits do the work that individual garments had to do in the past. Even so, many swimsuits, especially for the not-so-perfect woman—a category that includes almost everyone over the age of twenty—have internal panels that control and smooth and bras that shape and support. How many women would dare to wear one that lacked these improvements? A Speedo leaves little to either the imagination or the ego.

Few women—the very young, some of the outdoor-oriented, the dress reformers—refused to wear corsets, or, to be more specific, considered leaving them off. Ladies wore corsets. Nineteenth-century society drew a sharp line between the acceptability of wearing corsets and the dubious practice of tight lacing, a distinction often lost to later generations. The former was a routine part of women's clothing, the latter a focus of crusading reformers. The ambivalence towards corsets may be seen in *The Perfect Woman*, a house, family, and beauty care book of 1901, which featured an article on "Sallow Faces and Deformed Figures." In it was a list of "Madame Yale's . . . corset crimes against beauty." This list included everything from red noses and general feebleness to stupidity, wrinkles, and clumsiness, all brought on by the damnable corset. But eight pages later an inserted photo of a "Brunette—A Type of Beauty" depicted a soulful but sturdy young woman dressed in the height of the period's fashion, with prominent bosom and voluptuous hips separated by an amazingly delicate waist, narrow and curved as only a corset could make it.[21] So much for the list.

In short, there is no doubt that swimming corsets were worn. Indeed, *The Delineator*, as early as 1890, in describing its new pattern for a bathing corset, informs readers that this item fills a "a want that had long been experienced by fastidious bathers." The magazine suggests a variety of suitable cotton fabrics, "drilling, coutille, jean, sateen," and adds, "[the corset] is adjusted by gores and stiffened by whalebones."[22] Lighter in weight and less rigidly shaped than ordinary corsets, they were often advertised in the back of women's magazines of the time.

The bathing suit by century's end had begun to follow the lead of the English model, similar to the American one in every respect but without a skirt. The same jersey fabric used in tennis dresses at the time was also applied to swimwear. Its advantages of flexibility and stretch were obvious for use in sport clothing. By 1886 it was being used in "bathing jerseys," or form-fitting tunic tops, worn belted, which fell to cover the hips. These were paired with knee-length trunks and stockings.[23] Little change seems to have occurred in the popular swimming clothing for the next thirty or more years. *The Perfect Woman* illustrated one suit in a natty sailor-collar style. But even though this book was published in the Midwest, the illustration is in all likelihood English,[24] first because the subject's suit has no skirt (even though the swimmer is about to be swathed completely in a vast blanket, and so will maintain her proper decorum) but also, even more important, because she wears no stockings. Most American women, even children, always did. The clincher, though, is that all the background figures are women. By this time in the United States, as we have seen, men and women mingled at the beach. A second woman, looking every inch the perfect servant, complete with her encompassing apron and her tidy little bonnet, helps her poised mistress as she emerges from the water. Although the "servant" may simply be an attendant at a resort, somehow the image just *looks* British.

Borrowed images notwithstanding, *Harper's Bazar* stated with its customary authority in July 1897 that "American women certainly can take the lead in their designs for bathing suits, and they do not depend in any degree upon foreign fashion plates." Following up on their advice of a year earlier, the editors spent considerable time assessing the merits of various materials, stating that "flannel possesses many of the qualities that make serge desirable, but does not keep its color so well, and looks heavy and coarser." As to the question of stockings, they allowed no possible discussion. "It is not necessary on most beaches in this country," they said, "to wear bathing shoes." As a result, "bathing stockings are consequently universally worn." Apparently, since stockings stretched and spread, many women tried to put a sole inside. But, the magazine decreed, "this makes them clumsy." Once again, *Harper's* advised its readers to buy a "size too small and not elastic. Of course," the writer admitted, "they soon wear out, but the expense is one of the points to be faced if one wishes to be well turned out. It is a great mistake to buy cheap thin stockings. Heavy ribbed silk, or silk and wool, is the best, as they keep their shape longer and prevent the foot from spreading. Black stockings are always worn in preference to any others. They are most becoming and least conspicuous. They must be long enough to garter well above the knees, and ribbed are better than plain."[25] So once again, even with clothing for bathing, we see the acknowledgment that "being well turned out" was the primary consideration.

By the 1890s, though, more women were actually swimming, and therefore looking for more practical clothing to wear while doing it. J. Parmly Paret makes this perfectly clear in his 1901 *Woman's Book of Sports.* "Nothing tight should be worn for swimming, no matter how fashionable a dress may be for bathing," he declared. "The exercise requires the greatest freedom, and a swimming costume should never include corsets, tight sleeves, or a skirt below the knees. The freedom of the shoulders is the most important of all, but anything tight around the body interferes with the breathing and the muscles of the back, while a long skirt—even one a few inches below the knees—binds the legs constantly in making their strokes."[26] How far to have come, in the case of the corset at least, in five years. But notice that even Paret did not advise leaving the skirt off altogether. On the contrary, and surprisingly, he recommended a heavy knee-length sailor dress over tights. The differences between requirement and recommendation are often startling, and indicate perhaps more graphically than anything else just where the divide lay between common sense and custom. Perhaps the function of the clothing had diverged between swimming and bathing, but the look and weight of the outfits remained the same. In America, both were skirted.

A picture of Coney Island bathing beauties from 1897 indicates where the cutting edge of fashion was headed: all five beauties are dressed in short (mid-thigh) sleeveless or capped-sleeve dresses with bloomers of the same length, frilled and matching the dress. Their stockings are long and of various colors, and they wear different styles of shoes, from boots to slippers with criss-cross-tied ribbons climbing the calf to the knee. Clearly, these young women are "fast," "racy," not entirely genteel, perched as they were in a chorus-line pose, bent from the waist and holding their skirts up in the back to reveal their bloomers like so many cancan girls. One can assert with little fear of contradiction that they had no intention of leaving the beach for the more athletic adventures the water offered.

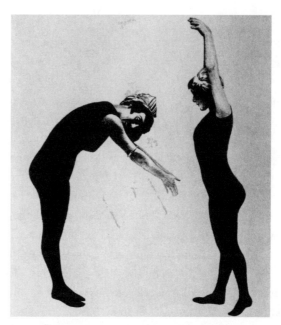

Annette Kellerman in her gymnasium-inspired swimsuit.
Ladies' Home Journal, August 1910.

Men, meanwhile, wore a one-piece knitted suit with a short sleeve or none at all, and short legs that stopped just above the knee. Englishwomen now wore something like this costume for swimming, but such a garment was still considered shocking in America. When the Australian Annette Kellerman, "the most famous diver and swimmer in the world," visited the United States in 1910, she wore a daring interpretation of this suit, one that actually bore a stronger resemblance to men's gym wear of the time than to men's bathing suits, since it borrowed the footed tights, small sleeves, modest scooped neck, and form-fitting torso typical of men's gymnastic.[27] Kellerman appeared in this costume (in the same pose as the Coney Island girls, it must be admitted) in her article "Why and How Girls Should Swim," featured in the *Ladies' Home Journal* for August 1910. Her dress may have been slightly scandalous, but her comments are of interest. "It is . . . timidity that keeps so many women in this country from learning to swim," she observed, "and so it has been considered a sport rather for boys than for girls."[28] Years later, in 1918, Kellerman wrote: "I am certain there isn't a single reason under the sun why everybody should not wear lightweight suits. Anyone who persuades you to wear the heavy skirty kind is endangering your life."[29]

Nevertheless, the "heavy skirty kind" continued to be worn well into the 1920s. Of course, by that time it had been updated with the flapper's dropped waist, but it still called for stockings and gaitered boots. Not everybody went all the way, however. My mother recalled her own experience, fixed in her memory to the year the family purchased a summer cottage, 1922, but continuing over the next couple of years while she was in high school. She and her best friend

> made our own bathing suits. They were navy blue, sort of a mercerized material, smooth, but not like sateen. They had yellow appliques; I'm sure they were sateen. My, we were pleased with ourselves.
>
> Mine had a sort of long top with a belt, cap sleeves, a modest boat neck, no fastenings. The bloomers had elastic around the waist and elastic around the knees. They were separate from the tunic. In our modesty we wore them below our knees. No, I don't think we wore stockings. We felt no embarrassment—there were no people around.[30]

In 1925 she was photographed wearing a two-piece black wool knit bathing suit with a long tunic over fitted pants covering the thighs, both hitting just above the knees. It was V-necked and sleeveless, buttoned at the shoulder, and trimmed with an edging of a different color, probably matching the wide double stripe across the bosom. She stands in the water with two men, one her father. Both wear essentially the male version of her suit, but notably the legs on their suits are considerably shorter than hers, cropped at upper mid-thigh. My mother mentioned an interesting offshoot of this new, more body-baring style. For the first time, she said, she and many other women of the period had to worry about shaving their underarms and legs. "It was a problem," she admitted. "Creams—in the ads they were perfection, and in reality, they weren't." She solved it by borrowing her father's razor, perhaps an early daughter to do so but certainly not the last.

Probably the single factor that most affected swimwear after the 1920s was the one thing that had nothing to do with swimming: the increased acceptance, indeed the rage, for tanned skin. Coco Chanel is said to have been among the first to introduce the look, but American expatriates of the Jazz Age, such as the splendidly elegant socialites Sarah and Gerald Murphy, who lived in the south of France, also helped the fashion along. Until the 1920s, women had worked assiduously to maintain their pale, freckle-free complexions. But the combination of a new awareness of leisure time, the much wider availability of motor cars after the introduction of Henry Ford's model T in 1908, easier access to beaches, the growth of Florida as a resort destination, the California boom in general and Hollywood movies in particular, and the daring increase in individual freedom after World War I all worked together to encourage people to uncover in the warmth of the postwar sunshine. Thus, clothing for resort wear, so closely related to swimwear, bared the skin for the first time outside of a competitive sport venue. It ushered in the fashion for bare arms, bare backs, and décolletage. For the first time, evening wear followed sport wear.

Perhaps the last element to catch up with the trend, more relevant to swimming than to bathing, was fabric. The same problems women faced when they first chose to dip themselves in water in public still remained. Although by 1928 the suits had more or less merged into a shorts/tunic style, evolving by the very early 1930s into a one-piece version with briefs instead of distinct legs, the material was still usually wool knit, often very heavy. Every now and then a heavy cotton knit was an alternative, but generally the suits were made of wool.[31] Cotton would soak up the water and drag down. If anything, wool shrank. This led to a frequent problem: the wool tended to felt, or become thick and matted, making the suit even stiffer and less comfortable than before. One woman recalled that these suits were attractive when dry but were "stretchy, saggy, itchy, and smelled of wet wool" when wet. At the beach, wool had the additional disadvantage of attracting and holding sand, making it even more uncomfortable.[32] A competitive swimmer in the 1920s and 1930s, the daughter of a well-known swim coach, remembered:

> In 1930 we still trained in that old smelly wool suit. But we competed in a black cotton suit that was lighter weight, but didn't give at all in the water. Then, in 1936, I got my first black chiffon suit. It was the fastest suit made then and I remember how expensive it was—$28, and in those days, you could feed a whole family for $15 a week.

It was terrible, that suit. People always asked me why I never went in for competitive swimming and I've always told them it was *because* of that awful black suit. It was the most unattractive thing; it hung like a chemise with no fit at all. If you had boobies, the suit flattened them down like two peas on an ironing board. At the widest point of your hips, about four inches down from the navel, it had this six-inch skirt attached. Just where you didn't need a line. And wet? It was the most revealing and clinging suit—you could see everything! The swimmers had people around them to bring them towels when they climbed out of the pool. Towels to hide in, not to dry with.[33]

But the hated, revealing silk shaved precious seconds from competition time, and so it was worn through the 1930s. Throughout the decade designers and swimmers made various attempts to create suits that were both fashionable and functional, including an all-rubber model demonstrated by leading swimmers, including Esther Williams, at the Los Angeles Coliseum. Alas, that one "split right down the front from the water pressure" at the first dive into the pool.[34] The designers, though momentarily dismayed, sensed they were on the right track, and eventually they got it right. In 1934 *Harper's Bazaar* advertised swimming suits made from a new thread, Lastex, which consisted of an elastic rubber core covered by cotton, rayon, or some other fiber—certainly a much more practical use of rubber than the sheet variety.[35] The post–World War II combination of Lastex yarn and nylon, perfected through the war effort, led the world into the era of fashionable, speed-enhancing swimwear for women. It fit better, it looked better, and it made smaller and closer-fitting suits possible even for women who didn't want to swim at all but just wanted to lie on the beach, get a suntan, and look good, as their grandmothers had done at the turn of the century in their modest bathing dresses.

The evolution has continued since then. Speedo introduced its revolutionary suits at the 1956 Melbourne Olympics, providing respite for a few years until the East German team wore a new "skirtless, second-skin" Lycra suit at the world championship games in Belgrade in the early 1970s. With each upgrade in design (usually tied to innovations in textiles and fibers), world speed records are smashed. In the 1970s, female competitors suggested that they be allowed to compete nude: the East German team, for example, formally requested permission for the 1976 Olympics. Both coaches and swimmers agreed that the competitors would swim faster if they were allowed to do so: "Girls with flat chests can make better times naked, no question about it," commented an Olympic coach. Although their very request tells us how far the world had come by then, at least some traditions of history held sway. The women were turned down because of "the spectator problem."[36] The next best thing to nudity, the suits of today have little drag, clinging so close to the body as to cover only the characteristics of sex while leaving everything else bare. It has been said that the social mores of America may be traced in the development of bathing suit styles—that they show the complete emancipation of women. Or, as the swimmer Joan Ryan says, echoing James Laver: "Almost, but not quite. Not until we swim in our birthday suits will the emancipation be complete."[37]

It seems the uneasy alliance between practicality and modesty is still with us. The swimsuits of today are the most revealing in history, baring pubic and buttock areas as never before. Yet women in America may still be arrested for baring their breasts on public beaches, and indeed, most would not want to, even if our European sisters might regard us as prudes for preferring to keep covered. The issue of the definition of freedom arises at this point. It is true that the body has complete mobility in these suits, since the idea of confinement in such wisps of fabric verges on the ridiculous. But though modesty no longer plays the role it once did, embarrassment now finds its outlet in the problem of body hair. Current designs force women to shave portions of their anatomy as never before, in places they might not have dreamed of a generation ago. A young woman emerging from sleeves for the first time in the early 1920s borrowed her father's razor to shave her underarms. Now there are creams and devices of astonishing array just to get the bikini line under control, and even to reduce hip and thigh cellulite, whatever that may be. Although fashions change, and in the past decade men too have begun to shave portions of their below-the-chin anatomy (their chests as much as anything, but backs are certainly part of the general anti-hair cleanup), men are regarded as attractive with hairy bodies. Women are not. It would seem that women are still slaves to beauty. And until women feel comfortable appearing in public with bodies that are free and natural, with hair and all, they will never experience the freedom men claim unthinkingly as their right.[38]

The development of clothing for water activities over the past 150 years has been intimately connected to modesty standards for women, and hence, broadly speaking, to gender expectations and the mores of each subsequent generation. Because of "the spectator problem" and the nature of wet fabric clinging to the human body, particular care has been taken in the design of the garments to provide opaque and often figure-concealing solutions. (Even today, the older you become, the more pressing the awareness of these problems.) Once again, we see that the gender context changed the nature of the clothing, for if women participated in the activities in a private, single-sex environment, their clothing allowed greater freedom from restraint, in terms of both prudery and movement. But the guidelines become hazy here because of the overlapping uses of the clothing—for bathing and sunbathing on the one hand and for active swimming on the other. When the strict separation of private and public is in place, represented by competitive swimming as opposed to sunbathing and dipping, the distinction is much clearer, at least during the years I concentrate on in this book. Only after the Second World War did the two functions successfully merge into a widely used, effective, and fashionable suit.

Women's interest first in swimming and bathing, then in water sports, grew slowly over a long period of time. Even so, what probably had the greatest impact was the acceptance of women's swimming and diving competitions in the Olympic Games. This too took a long time to gain ground, and it is to that story that we now turn. It represents in microcosm the struggles women faced in being accepted in competitive sports in general.

WOMEN ENTER THE *Olympics*

A Sleeker Swimsuit

SO FAR WE HAVE LOOKED AT THE LONG, SLOW GROWTH OF WOMEN'S involvement in sporting activities. Clothes certainly played their part. But nowhere is their influence more evident than in the Olympic Games. And nowhere else can we see quite so clearly the position of women at the end of the nineteenth century and the beginning of the twentieth, no matter what the trends of the previous half century might suggest. Anyone living today within reach of TV knows how important new developments in textile and clothing designs are for the success of athletes competing in the Games. We saw in the 2002 Winter Olympics in Salt Lake City the skintight racing suits worn by men and women alike, sleek and aerodynamic, capable of shaving precious milliseconds off time. That they enhanced beautiful bodies was almost an afterthought, although I'm sure no one who watched failed to enjoy that aspect of the new designs. We have taken technological advances and used them to serve speed as their products wrap bodies in garments that would have been unthinkable even a generation ago.[1] Hand in hand with this development has been the equally stunning acceptance of women as competitors, as athletes. Although women's competition became a media event as early as the 1996 Summer Games, when women were hailed as the stars who would outshine the men, it took a century to achieve this equality.[2]

In the beginning, in keeping with the ancient Greek tradition, the modern Olympic Games were all male. Only gradually over the course of the twentieth century did women enter the competition. Yet in the paeans to women's strength and athleticism that filled the popular press prior to the Centennial Games in 1996, the question of women's rare appearances during the first twenty-four years, from 1896 to 1920, was never raised. The total number of female participants in those first six Games amounted to less than 2 percent of the entire field.[3] Even at the turn of the present century, women's involvement is still little better than 35 percent. Why has this been so?

In our own time, articles in the popular press calculated to generate female pride often feature beauty, appearance, and the aesthetics of women's bodies in sport rather than women's athletic accomplishments. For women, whose worth until very recently was measured by their value as wives, mothers, and keepers of the hearth, beauty and appearance have always been used as currency to achieve a better position. At the beginning of the twentieth century, appeals to these qualities were used as well to keep women from participating in competitive sports. It will come as no surprise that clothing was, too. By being prohibited from wearing functional clothing appropriate for specific sports, American women were literally prevented from entering events, let alone excelling in them. This chapter, then, is a brief history of American women's progress towards overcoming the societal restraints that severely limited their participation in the early Olympic Games. It is a story that sports historians and journalists alike have largely ignored.[4] In no small measure it revolves around clothing. And ultimately it centers more specifically on swimwear than on any other kinds of dress.

Baron Pierre de Coubertin first publicly proposed the modern Olympics in 1892 and spent the next three years gathering support for his idea. When he first dreamed of a rebirth of the Olympic Games, it never entered his mind that women might want to participate. His beliefs were quite the opposite. "Women have but one task," he said, "that of crowning the winner with garlands."[5] As late as 1912 he wrote, "The Olympic Games . . . [are] the solemn and periodic exaltation of male athleticism with internationalism as a base, loyalty as a means, art for its setting, and female applause as reward."[6] Even when he traveled to the United States in 1889 and visited colleges offering women's physical exercise programs, such as Wellesley and the University of California at Berkeley, his attitude was decidedly patronizing. "Americans find that women, too, have the right to physical exercises," he said. "And why not? Women need natural movements in the out-of-doors as much as men do."[7] His own writing expresses his views of women succinctly. "Women have probably proved that they are up to par with almost all the exploits to which men are accustomed," he wrote in 1902, "but they have not been able to establish that in doing so, they have remained faithful to the necessary conditions of their existence and obedient to the laws of nature." Furthermore, "the French, by heredity, by disposition, by taste, are opposed to the idea of the apparent equality of the two sexes. They will accept the principle of real equality as long as it does not display itself too boisterously in the open, and that, in the expression it takes, it will not shock their deep-rooted traditions."[8]

Clearly, to Coubertin gender was destiny. The very idea of equality for women countered everything the Frenchman believed in. And of course he was not alone. In the late nineteenth century, when societal expectations for women were still largely limited to home and family, Coubertin merely represented his time and place, his sex, and the general expectations of his peers. Indeed, he was reputed to hate the sight of women sweating, involved in violent effort, since it killed their mystery and reduced them to "painful grins that give them sexless faces and bodies."[9] As a result, there was not one woman among the 311 athletes who participated in the first modern Olympics, held in Athens in 1896.[10]

So strong was Coubertin's influence that the second Games, held in 1900, were in Coubertin's own city, Paris, rather than once again in Athens, as the Greeks had wanted. Here, in spite of his strongly held beliefs, we see the first inroads in the tentative introduction of women into certain events. The Paris Games drew 1,330 athletes, a thousand more than four years earlier in Athens. Of these, twelve were women—and it seems that even this was a fluke. No one can say exactly how they got in. Apparently, no records survive. Probably, however, the key lies in the haphazard administration of the Paris Games, held to coincide with the Paris Exposition of 1900.[11] Coubertin believed that the Games would be the capstone of that world's fair, captivating the throngs who attended it as the earlier games had enthralled the audience in Athens. Thus, he was willing to turn the planning over to the Exposition committee. But these bureaucrats, who knew and cared nothing about sports, allowed the Games to become little more than a sideshow to the Exposition. The events dragged on for four to five months and were so poorly organized that several athletes who participated were not even aware that they were competing in the Olympics. In fact, the word "Olympics" never appeared in the official program.[12] In all likelihood, with the Games out of Coubertin's control and the general shambles that ensued, the twelve women were either ignored or overlooked.

Even so, it is hard to imagine what it would have been like to be one of those twelve. Most of the other athletes, and certainly most of the officials, would have shared Coubertin's views. Nonetheless, twelve women, representing Great Britain, France, Switzerland, Bohemia, and the United States, competed in golf and tennis. Margaret Abbott, age twenty-two, a five-foot-eleven socialite from the Chicago Golf Club who was studying art in Paris at the time, entered the nine-hole golf tournament at Compiègne and won. Later, she was credited with being the first American woman to win an Olympic medal, a gold, although in reality all she actually received was a ladylike gold-trimmed porcelain bowl.[13] Somewhat surprisingly, Margaret Abbott's mother, a "noted novelist and editor," also competed— possibly the first and last mother-daughter combination ever to do so. Abbott, in a graceful comment that sheds light on the quality of play, later claimed that she had won only because her French competitors "apparently misunderstood the nature of the game and turned up to play in high heels and tight skirts." An extant photograph of the game reveals hatted, long-sleeved, and long-skirted women, golf clubs gripped and in action. Interestingly, Abbott's comment emphasized the tightness of the dress, not its length.[14] One thing remains clear, though: the women competing were accorded neither team status, uniforms, nor any other kind of recognition by their respective Olympic committees; certainly the Abbotts were ignored by the American Olympic Committee (AOC).[15]

As we have seen, even by the turn of the century, women could not go out in public to participate in any sports activity with men while wearing anything but the traditional long skirt, shortened perhaps four to six inches to permit easier play. No surprise, then, that England's Charlotte Cooper, the first woman to win an official Olympic gold medal, is shown in a photograph, her hair in a perfect pompadour, wearing the typical stiff, high-collared

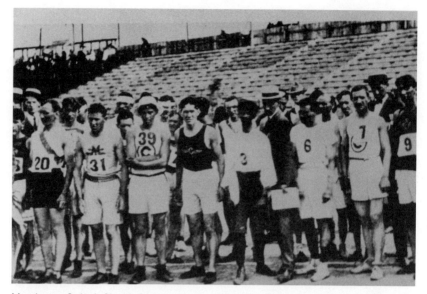

Marathoners, St. Louis Olympic Games, 1904. Shorts and tank tops contrast sharply with the dragging skirts and high stiff collars women wore for sports. Courtesy of United States Olympic Committee.

shirtwaist and fitted-at-the-hip, gored skirt, tightly corseted, and belted at her narrow waist, displaying her tennis racquet to the photographer. A startled young Frenchman in Paris wrote to a friend after catching some of the events: "Brace yourself, my friend, women have participated in these games. . . . Our sportswomen were clad in white, elegant, pretty, and the racket they held in their hands did not just caress the ball! Their ardor and their endurance have astonished me!"[16] Men by contrast, bared their bodies far more, wearing fitted tank tops and narrow, above-the-knee shorts. The contrast in standards—and appearance—is evident.

The 1904 Games, held in St. Louis, were smaller, with only 617 athletes altogether, eight of whom were women. All eight were archers, a sport new to the Olympics, and all were American.[17] Indeed, most of the athletes were American. These Games, like the previous ones, were held to coincide with the St. Louis World's Fair, and resulted in much the same debacle as the Paris Games.

In 1904 the American Olympic Committee was closely aligned with the Amateur Athletic Union. The AAU secretary, James E. Sullivan, chaired the organizing committees for both the all-male 1896 Athens team and the St. Louis Games. He shared Coubertin's views of women in sports, agreeing that participation was unwomanly, that women should not strain to excel, and that they certainly should not wear clothing that came above the ankle in order to play sports. Hence, tennis, golf, and archery were the only events possible for women, since these required only subtle modifications of the current fashionable dress. He was typical of his time, and was supported by all the men involved in the American Olympics movement and in sports generally. Even one of the more progressive men involved in sport and athletic pursuits, Luther Harvey Gulick, proposed in 1906 that "athletics for women should for the present be restricted to sport within the school; that they should be used for recreation and pleasure; that the strenuous training of teams tends to be injurious to both body and mind; that public, general competition emphasizes qualities that are on the whole unnecessary and undesirable. Let us then have athletics for recreation, but not for serious, public competition."[18] One can only imagine what the more conservative leaders in America thought. But their attitudes were put into action when it came to awards: women received diplomas for their successes; men won medals.[19]

Fortunately, somewhat more enlightened views prevailed abroad. The 1908 London Olympics admitted women in tennis, figure skating, and archery, which had replaced golf in 1904. Thirty-six out of 2,020 participants were women, most of them from the British Isles.[20] None was American. What caught the eye of the British press, though, were the Scandinavian women's gymnastic demonstration teams, who, though not strictly Olympians, certainly drew attention to women's athleticism. The *London Daily Telegraph* focused particularly on the Danish team, reporting that twenty or more Danish "ladies in neat gymnastic costume [were] instantly appreciated by the multitude, who gave vent to their admiration by prolonged applause." The reporter gave a rare description of their uniforms, thereby telling us by its very inclusion just how unusual the clothing was: "The presence of their party of ladies in white serge gymnastic costumes and pale brown stockings, without shoes, would of itself have arrested the multitude."[21] No question about that: those pale brown stockings no doubt gave the appearance of bare legs to that appreciative multitude.

These toeholds, small though they seem, and not part of the Olympic events proper, represented the beginnings of change. The Games held in

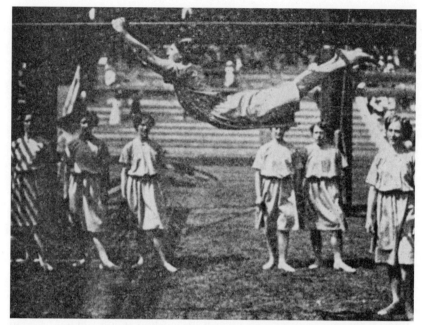

Finnish gymnasts, 1912 Olympics in Stockholm. The loose, unstructured, and unconfining dress, worn over bare legs and feet, was years ahead of its time. Fred Eugene Leonard, *History of Physical Education*, 1923.

Stockholm in 1912 reflected the more liberal attitudes of the Scandinavian countries, which had a strong history of women's participation in physical exercise.[22] Once again, Denmark and Finland, as well as the other Scandinavian countries, sent gymnastic teams to Stockholm. The Danes wore the same general style of costume they had worn in London four years before: a garment based on the baggy bloomer, American-style gymnastic suit. But the Finns' dress was nothing short of astonishing in such a venue. It was skirted, knee-length, short-sleeved, probably based on a costume for dance, and the women were bare-legged and barefoot—altogether remarkable for 1912. (I had a dress almost like it in the 1960s.)[23]

Members of the International Olympics Committee voted in their Luxembourg meeting in 1910 to introduce an even greater innovation at the Stockholm Olympics, one that would have lasting consequences: they agreed to include swimming events for women. The first was the women's 100-meter freestyle race.[24] At this point we should pause to remember how far women's swimming and bathing dress had developed. Modesty had always taken precedence over common sense, but by the twentieth century, there was a marked distinction between the two and the clothing each supported. As we saw in Annette Kellerman's comments, made in 1910, American women by and large did not know how to swim. And the modesty factor was an even bigger problem in the United States than in Europe or Great Britain. Americans were far more prudish than their counterparts elsewhere, and the issue of immodesty was one of the chief arguments against allowing American women to enter competitions, especially in water sports. Besides, the U.S. Olympic Committee had voted down women's participation. So once again, in the 1912 Stockholm Olympics, American women did not participate.[25]

Some fifty-five others did, though, forty-one of them swimmers representing ten countries.[26] Among these were English swimmers and, most visibly, two Australians, Fanny Durack and Wilhemina (Mina) Wylie. It was they who won the gold and silver individual medals. They too had a difficult time in their struggle to convince authorities that they were worthy of representing their country in the Olympics. Much of the concern in Australia, as in America, centered on the question of modesty and morality, which ultimately came down to the symbol of costume suitable for mixed company. Finally, the young women were grudgingly accepted as part of the Australasian team, but only on the condition that they raise their own travel and support money. Australia refused to sponsor them, pleading insufficient funds even for all the men going.

The women's fight against a strong conservative tradition, represented, paradoxically, by Rose Scott, a powerfully militant "old" woman, makes a fascinating story. Scott's Victorian roots undergirded her "heavy sense of prudishness," as is most evident in the following anecdote: determined to protect the virtue of the young women swimmers, she arranged for a brass band to perform during a meet in Australia but made sure to hire one whose players were all blind. It seems odd, then, that Rose Scott is known as a great defender of women's rights, and "the mother of suffrage" in New South Wales. Apparently she was as socially conservative as she was politically liberal. She made her position perfectly clear: "We are essentially a clothes-wearing people. . . . It is immodest for ladies to appear on open beaches amongst men in attire so scant that they would be ashamed to wear the same dress in their own drawing rooms." Needless to say, she brought this view to bear against Durack and Wiley. Luckily for the swimmers, many in Australia supported them, though acknowledging the problem of dress. One writer to the *Daily Telegraph* suggested a solution: the swimmers "should not mix with the audience, and should wear long coats over their costumes whenever they were out of the water."[27]

What did the 1912 swimsuits look like? And how revealing were they? What was causing all the concern among the sponsors? Were these still the multilayered costumes of the turn of the century, or had the women athletes devised new, more efficient swimwear to better meet the needs of competitive swimming? Perhaps it is helpful to look back at that other famous Australian swimmer, Annette Kellerman, in order to answer those questions. She had made a career of traveling and demonstrating her scandalous new suit, based on men's gym wear, and of inspiring girls and women to swim. The Western world knew her and her costume. The two girls from New South Wales could scarcely have avoided knowing of her. Certainly she influenced many, and her crusade to educate women about the pleasure of swimming must have helped Fanny and Mina's cause. But perhaps her influence was in the deed, not the dress. Photographs of their costumes make it clear that these two women chose not to copy Kellerman's style. They followed other swimmers instead—not women but men.

A photograph exists of a 1900 Olympics swimmer, the Australian Freddie Lane, wearing a typical male racing suit of the day. It is one-piece with a tank top, and cut high at the hip to bare almost the entire leg. Other photos, of Duke Kahanamoku from Hawaii, the U.S. champion in 1912, and of the four-man Australasian freestyle swim team at the Stockholm Olympics, all show versions of the same suit. Two or three of these suits, though dark in tone, look surprisingly sheer, to the point where nipples and other details of the body show through. It is scarcely surprising, then, that underneath their suits and quite visible, the swimmers wore a bikini-like bottom, known as an "athletes'."[28] Certainly more startling for 1912, though, is a photograph of American Olympic swimmers stripped down for action, wearing this scanty garment only. The modest, covering suit worn for competition is nowhere in sight. The fabric out of which the suits were made remains a mystery. They stretch to fit and define the body, so clearly are some kind of knit, but it is hard to state with any certainty what the fiber

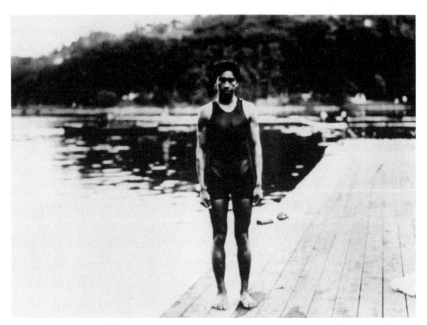

Duke Kahanamoku, U.S. Olympic champion, 1912, in his silky suit that reveals bikini-like undershorts. Courtesy of United States Olympic Committee.

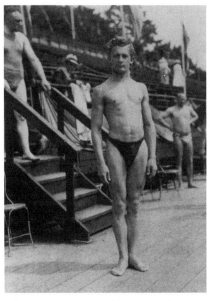

U.S. swimmer at the 1912 Olympics wearing an "athletes'" without the covering suit. Courtesy of United States Olympic Committee.

actually was. My own guess for the sheerer ones would be a silk knit, and for the others cotton, or possibly wool. Silk swimming suits for racing existed later, in the late 1920s and early 1930s, and were worn in competition then, but I have never been able to find proof that silk, let alone silk knit, was used for swimming as early as the 1910s. Certainly, cotton knit was used in England and elsewhere for men's swimsuits as early as the end of the nineteenth century.[29] Careful study of these 1912 photographs, however, suggests a finer, sheerer, and silkier fabric than cotton. Duke Kahanamoku's suit fits him perfectly, etching every muscle and detail of his body, highlighting it with a kind of sheen, and clearly revealing the bikini-style brief underneath. The fabric looks very different from the opaque suit worn by at least one of the Australasian swimmers, or the semi-opaque suit worn by one of his teammates.

The two Australian women posed for the photographer in female versions of the same style, but very likely theirs were made from cotton or wool knit, to judge by the drape and opacity. Each found a different solution to the modesty problem. Mina Wylie's suit has longer legs, fitting tightly to within a few inches above her knees. Hers also had an extra layer in the form of a bikini brief underneath the lightweight, almost certainly cotton outer suit, as did Duke Kahanamoku's. Fanny Durack, by contrast, wears her extra layer on top, as a hip-length tunic over shorter pants, both clearly wool. Fanny was the outstanding female swimmer of that Olympics, and interestingly, it was her swimsuit that became the standard well into the 1930s, in no small part, one imagines, because it was considerably more becoming than Mina's.[30] It is the swimsuit my own mother wore over a decade later in 1925 at the beach.

The English women's 100-meter relay team offers interesting early versions of the racing suit as well. In a 1912 photograph each of the four members wears a slightly different style, from the almost opaque to the startlingly sheer. All four appear to be wearing the bikini-style briefs underneath, which are more clearly visible on some than on others, as are other details, such as the breasts. The fabric in all four suits seems to be a cotton knit. But here we see a new addition: unlike the Australians (who were unsure that they would be allowed to go to Stockholm until the very last minute), the English swimmers display Union Jacks emblazoned on their swimsuit chests, announcing their nationality to the world; now, of course, this is a commonplace. The photograph also reveals each of the four looking supremely uncomfortable having her picture taken. Each stands soberly with arms firmly clasped across her chest, three of the four unwilling to meet the camera's eye, even though they had just won first place. So all those years of decorous modesty had apparently taken their toll, even among these pioneers of women's competition.

Back in the United States, the battle to allow women to compete was still going strong. James E. Sullivan, now the president of the AAU, maintained his iron control over amateur athletics in the United States. In 1913 he wrote a letter to the American Life Saving Society, which was planning schoolboy races in conjunction with women's swimming events. The letter, reprinted in the *New York Times*, reads, "Of course you know that the Amateur Athletic Union of the United States does not permit women or girls to be registered in any of its associations, and does not sanction open races for women in connection with Amateur Athletic Union events." Ida Schnall, the captain of the New York Female Giants baseball club, who had publicly expressed women's interest in the diving events at the Stockholm Olympics the year before, also used the *Times* to snap back: "[Sullivan] is always objecting, and never doing anything to help the cause along for a girls' AAU. He objects to a mild game of ball or any kind of athletics for girls. He objects to girls wearing a comfortable bathing suit. He objects to so many things that it gives me cause to think he must be very narrow minded and that we are in the last century."[31] Nevertheless, even in the face of rising opposition, Sullivan sent out a resolution to all AAU committee members to be voted on in January 1914. The wording almost guaranteed the results he was looking for: "Resolved: That the AAU does not and will not recognize the registration of women athletes and it is the sense of this committee that the rules were designatedly formed to include none but the male sex."[32] Only one committee member voted against it. So, women stayed out.

This was, however, a significant year for American female athletes, especially swimmers. Two things happened. First, that summer the Rye Beach Swimming Club in Westchester County, New York, helped the women determine to compete by holding a fifty-yard exhibition swimming race for women, thereby attracting attention to their cause. It was no small matter, because in doing so the club defied the AAU's stringent laws and jeopardized its membership in the New York Metropolitan Association of the AAU.

But the second event, and one that sped the process most significantly, was the death of James E. Sullivan in September 1914.[33] It is no coincidence that in November, the AAU governors voted to let women register for swimming. Committee members acknowledged that women would have been admitted much earlier had it not been for Sullivan, but none of them had dared to oppose him.

In speaking for the motion, a couple of members obliquely referred to the issue of dress, appearance, and modesty. Seward A. Simons of the Southern Pacific Association (California), in proposing the special legislation to allow women to compete, said, "I have never seen in any contest any act of immodesty that would bring the blush of shame to any man, mother, or child." Everett Brown of the Central Association also spoke in favor of the amendment, noting that "with the exception of France and the United States every member of the seventeen countries [of the International Amateur Athletic Federation] voted for the competition of women." Furthermore, "there was never a hint . . . of any immodesty or immorality and . . . absolutely [there was] the highest regard for women. I personally saw competitions at Stockholm and if there was any criticism there, it might have been brought about by foul minds."[34] The revealing character of the swimming costume, however, remained a stumbling block.

An incident that occurred the following year, 1915, tells the story best. A news item about a seventeen-year-old schoolgirl wearing a one-piece bathing suit drew the attention of a former AAU Board of Governors member. His indignation propelled him to criticize the "objectional features" of women's swimming generally and the teenager's "shocking" immodesty in particular. In reaction, he brought forward a motion to cancel women's competition altogether. But at the eleventh hour it was rejected, and women's involvement in amateur events was secured.[35]

No Olympics were held in 1916 because of World War I, but in 1917 the Women's Swimming Association of New York (WSANY) was founded and began training swimmers for competition. They experimented with lighter-weight clothing, trying to avoid the heavy wool suits that were reputed to gain an estimated forty pounds in the swimming of just one lap. That same year Ethelda Bleibtrey, the future Olympian, was arrested for "nude swimming" on New York's Manhattan Beach because she had taken off her shoes and stockings to swim bare-legged.[36] The publicity, her stubbornness, and the precedent set by the women swimmers in previous Olympics finally paid off, leading to the sanctioning of bare-legged swimming in the 1920 Olympics in Antwerp.

The Americans adopted swimsuits similar to those worn earlier by the Australians, as in the photograph of the prepubescent fourteen-year-old Aileen Riggin, who won the gold for springboard diving. In 1996 Riggin (later Soule), ninety years old and still swimming and writing, visited the U.S. Swimming Olympic trials. "I wrote down a list of 50 things that swimmers have today that we didn't," she noted, "everything from starting blocks to weights to suits. You should have seen our suits, with their little ruffled skirts. And they were made of *wool*. Imagine what wet wool feels like against your skin."[37] To judge by the photo of her in the official Report of the American Olympic Committee from the 1920 Antwerp Games, her memory served her well as to the wool suit, with its tight-fitting, hip-length tunic tank top covering the pants underneath, but it did not have the "little ruffled skirt" she remembered in 1996. Photos in the same report show "Four American Mermaids"[38] wearing suits identical to the American men's suits, in two different styles, one with a higher-cut neckline. Both styles are tank suits. All four look wet in the photos, and once again, it is difficult to identify the fabric, other than some sort of knit. Riggin's suit was definitely wool, and looks it in her photo; from the drape and wet shine on the bodies, the four "mermaids" seem to be wearing cotton suits. It is tempting to conclude, although no sources specify, that the divers' suits were wool but the racers' suits were cotton, since the latter would soak up less water to weigh the swimmer down. Suits for action swimming that year echoed the Olympic style, whether worn by other competitive swimmers or shown as advertisements in the popular press. Bathing dresses, however, were still the fashion-oriented "heavy, skirty kind" with the ruffled skirts, as Soule described, and would continue to be for another half decade.[39]

American women had won their battle—not the war, perhaps, but definitely the battle. With Sullivan dead, they finally could participate, and wear clothing designed to help them, not hold them back. As *The New York Times* reported in 1914, Sullivan had "opposed . . . women taking part in any event in which they could not wear long skirts."[40] But now, fully prepared and dressed to win, the American women swept the Olympic swim events in the 1920 Antwerp Games, with Ethelda Bleibtrey, bare-legged of

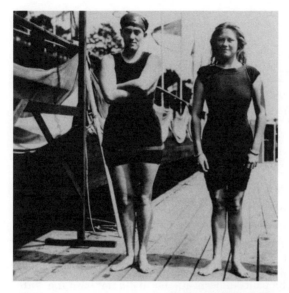

Australian swimmers Fanny Durack and Wilhemina Wylie. Note Durack's tunic top baring her shoulders, almost certainly of wool; Wylie's cotton suit has a hint of sleeves and reveals her "bikini" underneath. Courtesy of United States Olympic Committee.

Fourteen-year-old diver Aileen Riggin (left), and an Olympic rival beside her; both wear the knit wool tunic-top suit that was to become the classic 1920s swimsuit. Courtesy of United States Olympic Committee.

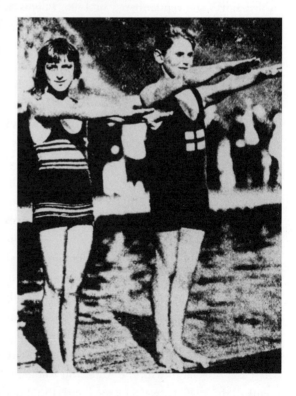

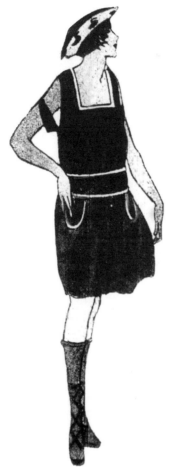

Stewart & Company advertisement, *New York Times*, July 4, 1920, showing "the heavy, skirty kind" of bathing dress, complete with all its accessories. In this ad, it is now referred to as a "bathing suit."

course, emerging a triple gold winner, the first American woman actually to receive a gold medal.[41]

Along with 2,543 men, 64 women were entered in the 1920 Games.[42] The *New York Times*, though it lauded Bleibtrey, never ran a single photo of her, certainly not in her bathing suit. It would seem that, even as late as 1920, "all the news that's fit to print" could not accommodate a photograph of an Olympic swimming medalist in what society still considered an immodest swimsuit. Even the language of the *Times* reveals the attitudes of the day:

Dateline Antwerp, Aug. 29 (Associated Press)

The American swimming team won the final of the 800-meter swimming relay here today, creating a new Olympic record of 10 minutes 4 2.5 seconds. The team was composed of [four men].

The final heat of the 400-meter relay swimming race for women was won by the American team. The American mermaids hung up a new Olympic record for the event, 5 minutes 11 4.5 seconds.[43]

The influence of the Women's Swimming Association of New York must not be undervalued. Almost all the swimmers who won in 1920 at Antwerp and 1924 in Paris were trained there, and most had joined in the first place to learn how to swim.[44] Mary Leigh, whose work has so informed most writers on women in the early Olympics, credits the Americans' "sensational new strides" during and after World War I to the "revolutionary" new "American crawl" as taught at the WSANY.[45] Harry Gordon, who fully understood the societal restraints under which the Australian women struggled, gave credit to the Australian crawl, overlooking the functional suits the swimmers wore. Clearly, it was the stroke that defeated the English swimmers in Stockholm in 1908, since all the women seem to have worn variations on the same suit. There is no doubt that the stroke, whether American or Australian, was a major factor in the emergence of women's competitive swimming, but its application must be paired with the new, sleeker suits to explain the emergence of women as swimming stars. Yet of all the sources on the history of women in the Olympics or in sports, only two, Paula Welch and Harold Lerch's *History of American Physical Education* as well as Gordon, specifically mention clothing or link the issue of clothing with women's participation in any way. Welch and Lerch attributed the long skirts to Sullivan's resistance, and Gordon, as we have seen, links the clothing to the mores of the time. But no one has drawn a specific causal relationship between the Americans' winning in 1920 and the dress they wore to do it.

To a historian of dress, it seems obvious that engagement in sports, certainly for American women, depended almost completely on clothing, first as a physical factor that hampered movement, and second as a societal factor that, for very different reasons, hampered participation. Although most universally, sports historians ignore the significance of clothing as a factor in the development of women's involvement in any athletic endeavor, without appropriately functional clothing, successful participation in the early days, as we have seen, was impossible. No amount of training in the crawl, whether Australian or American, would have helped a swimmer excel if she'd had to wear a suit that soaked up water, dragged against her progress, or pulled her under.

As an afterword to this story, it is interesting to note what has happened since 1920. From this account, it would seem that American women surmounted the barrier once and for all in those 1920 Olympic Games. Society's disapproval of women in sports, however, has been a long time dying. Just a few years later, in 1926, a German, Walter Kuhn, wrote about the ugliness of women straining and sweating for athletics: "And could such a woman see herself in the mirror, I believe she would consider very carefully whether or not she would continue such activities, because one cannot but agree that participation in contests results in a loss of femininity and therewith the finest that one esteems her." Thus, he concluded, it was a mistake to bring equality of the sexes into sports.[46]

The numbers seem to reflect this attitude. Even later in the century, men outnumbered women in the Olympics 4 to 1 until the late 1980s, when the ratio dropped to 3 to 1. In 1996, out of the 10,800 athletes who competed that summer, an estimated 3,800 were women, still maintaining approximately a 3-to-1 ratio.[47] In the Summer Games in Sydney in 2000, the numbers improved but did not reach 40 percent. And the press still reports on women's clothing and appearance. As Florence Griffith Joyner competed in every Olympiad from 1984 in Los Angeles to Atlanta in 1996, her clothing, her appearance, even her fingernails were fodder for comment. Although a few journalists mentioned the very brief, sleek swimsuits, reminiscent of those 1912 under-bikinis, that men such as Mark Spitz or Greg Louganis wore when they won their golds, their appearance failed to raise little more than eyebrows. By contrast, in April 1996 the women's track and field team at Florida State University won a meet but were disqualified because their uniform, with "bun hugger" bottoms, was judged unacceptable—too brief, too revealing.[48] And in Amherst, Massachusetts, perhaps one of the most liberal towns in the entire country, in the spring of 1996 two high-school-aged sisters received much local press, some of it startlingly negative, when they refused to play on the Amherst Regional High School lacrosse team because they were forced to wear kilts (a final remnant of Victorianism) instead of the more functional and gender-neutral shorts. Taking us full circle in regards to the initial issue of appearance, officials for the 1998 Winter Olympics complained that mixed-doubles luge was in jeopardy as a sport because no women were entered in it. They were discouraged "because two people lying on a sled don't look nice." As recently as the 2002 Salt Lake Games, the excuse for prohibiting women from competing in the ski jump was the same one that has been used for the past 150 years: that women's "delicate physiology" would be too shaken by the jarring of the landings (never mind that girls who live in the mountains have been ski jumping probably for as long as their brothers).[49] Given such stereotypes and criticism, women must still struggle to find roles—clothing—acceptable to themselves and to the people who set the rules.

In short, Coubertin's spirit remains alive and well. It is interesting to speculate whether the Games, now so keenly anticipated, would ever have come into existence without his obsession. But he resisted women's participation in athletics until his dying day. In 1934 he declared that "women will always be imperfect copies. There is nothing to learn from watching them; so those who assemble for this purpose have other things in mind."[50]

In this brief look at women's early participation in the Olympics, I have attempted to show some of the steps through which women finally achieved their goals of participation and success. Of course, this struggle did not take place in a vacuum, even in regard to clothing. The emergence of women's clothing for sports activities paralleled the loosening of boundaries that enclosed women's lives in the first decades of the twentieth century. Dress for women was changing significantly on all fronts, loosening cut, drape, fit, and underwear. But the Olympics, whose history has been well examined by many writers, have always provided a springboard for new ideas and designs for sleekness, speed, and success in a highly competitive world. Men have had an advantage from the start in being able to wear pared-down shorts and tank tops, body-hugging swimsuits, and lean, skin-baring outfits for individual events, all without social stigma. Women have had to work to gain their own lean, pared-down outfits that permit them to compete and to succeed. Interestingly, with the advanced stretch textiles available today, athletes are beginning to cover up again. Better yet, men and women are wearing much the same clothing to do the same jobs. The second skins they wear to compete once again shave valuable fractions of seconds off their time.

BICYCLING
AND THE
$\mathcal{B}$loomer

ON THE SURFACE OF IT, BECAUSE OF ITS SINGLE-MINDED IF SLOW DRIVE TO free the female body, clothing for swimming offered the greatest change in women's dress worn in public. As the early Olympic experiences show, however, the underlying demands of modesty—the need to cover limbs and the constancy of skirts prevailed even in that realm until the second decade of the twentieth century. Even then, although they were created for the specific purpose of competition, the streamlined new suits stirred up disquietude, ambivalence, and a certain amount of embarrassment. The task of that clothing was not easy. It had to break not only from the iron-bound restrictions caused by the clothing itself, but also from an outdated moral code enforcing puritanical standards of modesty. Different from swimming but with its own peculiar set of requirements, one last sporting pastime must be mentioned because of its importance in its own contemporary setting. That activity was bicycling. In its time, which in fact was relatively short—broadly speaking, from 1887 to 1903, with a fashionable peak from, roughly, 1895 to 1897—it took the nation by storm, generating untold numbers of articles in all kinds of the popular press. Commentaries and even entire magazines were devoted exclusively to it. Sports clubs and racing meets proliferated to respond to the demand. Clothing for both men and women was designed for it, and even today, over a hundred years later, the myth of the wholesale acceptance of the bicycle bloomer is still alive and well in costume histories. The bicycle bloomer may be said to be the first media creation of the modern era. That it existed cannot be denied; that it was worn much is another story entirely.

In order to understand where it stemmed from, we must first go back for a brief look at the dress reform movements that struggled throughout the last half of the nineteenth century, since they eventually had an impact on the clothing for cycling. Much has been written about dress reform by twentieth- and twenty-first-century authors, in part, perhaps, because they are struck by the realization that other women were willing to take on the struggle for sensible dress long before modern-day women had to tackle the problem.[1] Of course, every era has struggles of its own over the subject of clothing. Nonetheless, each generation happily embraces the fashion of its time, no matter how ridiculous it may come to look to that generation's daughters and granddaughters. The twentieth century, with its preference for physical comfort literally supported by stretchy manufactured fibers that became lighter and freer as the century grew old, particularly found the two previous centuries' clothing unfathomable—beautiful, but ferociously uncomfortable. So to find stalwart women swimming upstream in their search for sanity in dress offers us a glimmer of reason in the midst of convention. That is what the dress reformers, however difficult it was for them, and however unsuccessful they ultimately were, do for us: they give a promise of reason. We have had a tendency to enfold them into our free-breathing, gossamer-elastic underwear sisterhood as the pioneers they were, determined and righteous enough to insist on shorter skirts, lightweight corsets (or no corsets at all), and simple, unhooped and unbustled skirts—in fact, to embrace early versions of the kinds of clothes *we* wear. These, of course, were clothes that included some version of the trouser.

The dress reform movement began in the United States with the Turkish trouser outfit that Amelia Bloomer introduced to a wide and unwitting audience through her temperance publication *The Lily* in 1851. Called by a variety of names—including the "freedom dress" (the term preferred by women's rights advocates), the "American costume," and finally, lastingly, the "bloomer," its beginnings are clouded. Gayle Fischer gives as clear an explanation as it is possible to find, and sets it well within the framework of the utopian communities and water cures that abounded in the early nineteenth century.[2] One thing is evident: no matter what it was labeled, it had

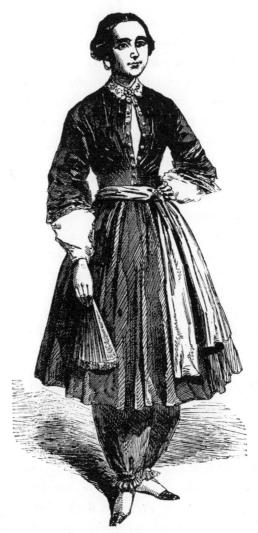

Amelia Bloomer wearing her "freedom dress," 1851. Library of Congress.

full trousers gathered at the ankle, which were more often than not referred to as Turkish. On top of those, women generally wore the fashions of their day, with a skirt cut off just below the knee. At least one version, however, a very early representation of Amelia Bloomer herself, shows an entire outfit that reflects Turkish origins. It consists of a fitted dress with open sleeves in the style of the time, buttoned from the waist down but left open in the bodice to show a full-sleeved blouse underneath, and a sash belt. Although it retains the silhouette of the early 1850s, the details are very much Middle Eastern.[3] Bloomer herself, writing in *The Lily*, suggested: "We would have the skirt reaching down to a little below the knee, and not made quite so full as is the present fashion. Underneath this skirt, trousers made moderately full."[4] But she makes no reference to Turkish dress at all. In another instance, an 1852 issue of *The Water-Cure Journal* published an illustration of an obviously Turkish costume, complete with a short-sleeved overdress worn over a long, straight-sleeved underblouse, both decorated, as well as the skirt of the overdress and the cuffs of the straight-legged pants, with embroidered motifs.[5] One wonders if the adaptation of a Middle Eastern style of dress was meant to lend an exotic aura to the outfit, one that might take away from the shock of the new, the shock of women wearing trousers. Perhaps the reformers reasoned that if it were foreign, it might be acceptable. If so, they were wrong. The costume was ridiculed widely by the national and international press, the church, and was even disdained by more conventional women (let alone men), who, it turned out, were far more numerous than the reformers in their own country.

Forty years later the Boston social reform publication *The Arena* devoted two issues to dress reform, one in 1892, the other the following year.[6] Amelia Bloomer had written an article for the *Ladies' Home Journal*, looking back at the furor caused by her "freedom dress." *The Arena* reprinted it in its entirety in 1893. In it, telling her own story as she remembered it, she stated that both Elizabeth Smith Miller and Miller's cousin Elizabeth Cady Stanton, then living in Seneca Falls and a neighbor of Mrs. Bloomer's, wore the garment before she herself did. Then in April 1851 her *Lily* article on her own adoption of the style was picked up by the *New York Tribune*, she recalled,

and made known to its thousands of readers . . . and from this it went from paper to paper throughout this country and countries abroad. I found myself noticed and pictured in many papers at home and abroad. I was praised and censured, glorified and ridiculed, until I stood in amazement at the furor I had wrought by my pen while sitting in my little office at home attending to my duties. . . .

It consisted of a skirt shortened to a few inches below the knees, and the substitution of trousers made of the same material as the dress. In other respects the dress was the same as worn by all women. At the outset, the trousers were full and baggy; but we improved upon them by making them narrower and gathered at the ankle, and finally by making them entirely plain and straight, falling to the shoe like the trousers of men.

To some extent, I think the style was adopted abroad, but not largely, or, for that matter, at home. . . . None of us [referring to other early women's rights activists, such as Lucy Stone and Elizabeth Cady Stanton] ever lectured on the dress question, or in any way introduced it into our lectures. We only wore it because we found it comfortable, convenient, safe, and tidy—with no thought for introducing a fashion, but with the wish that every woman would throw off the burden of clothes that was dragging her life out.[7]

Such a fond hope. Fashion, strong as ever, won the day. Stung by the devastating results of their attempt to adopt functional attire, women waited some twenty years before reintroducing the idea. This time, the thrust and direction came from England under the aegis of the Rational Dress Society, led by the stalwart Viscountess Harberton, who is credited with inventing "the divided skirt" sometime around 1876.[8] (It didn't hurt the movement that the Rational Dress Society was led by a titled lady.) The Americans followed her lead, climbing back on the battered reform bandwagon. By the 1870s, however, with experience their guide, those involved were well aware that if they were to succeed, some deference must be paid to fashion. As Abba Goold Woolson explained in her introduction to an 1873 published collection of five lectures titled *Dress-Reform*, the originators of the Bloomer had assumed that the great numbers of dissatisfied women who longed for more sensible clothing would adopt the new outfit, regardless of its source and configuration, and "make secure . . . its reign." Alas, she mourned, the women who stood behind it in principle lacked the courage to wear it in person, while

the majority of thoughtless women [held it as] an object of indifference or of ridicule. For them, nothing could be right which was not fashionable; and nothing could be fashionable which had not come from Paris. They were strengthened in their hostility by that half of humanity whose favor they chiefly sought, and who, as they had never experienced the miseries of the old attire, could never appreciate the comforts of the new. Men sneered at the costume without mercy, and branded it as hideous. As made and worn by many of its followers, it was certainly not beautiful: but had it been perfection itself, it would have utterly perished; for arrayed against it were the force of ignorance and of habit, and the persistent prejudices to which they give rise. Those who devised it had taken no pains to humor long-established tastes. . . . A few clung to it resolutely: but they learned at last that the mental discomfort it brought . . . outweighed the physical comfort it gave.[9]

Another twenty years passed, and *The Arena* still sang the same woeful song, albeit with a snappish edge: "If the Bloomer dress had come from a Paris milliner, it would have been welcomed in Boston, New York, and Philadelphia."[10] The prevailing notion of beauty—as we have seen, a factor in keeping women out of the earliest Olympics—played its role here as well. The anger and frustration the reformers lived with exploded in *The Arena*, caps, italics and all: "The women [of the 1860s] were beautiful in [hoop skirts], as they are *in anything which the majority of them wear*. . . . Were they beautiful? . . . They were frightful! and the fact is, women will wear anything under the sun that is fashionable; and THEIR WEARING IT *will, for the time, make it seem beautiful*."[11]

Even with the insights gained by the 1870s, the reformers had progressed little. By the 1890s, when the symposium reported in *The Arena* took place, women still struggled to create a worthy, accepted, functional costume. Again, those involved were leaders in the women's rights movement, and though vocal in their dismay and protest, they ultimately achieved as little immediate change in the area of dress reform as they did in the area of female enfranchisement.

Nonetheless, a growing number of influences helped renew the vigor of dress reform by the last decade of the century. The participants in the symposium gave credit over and over again to the increasing involvement of women's higher education and the need for women to dress comfortably when in competition with men on campuses. They expressed hope that with education, woman would "reach a plane where fashion will no longer enslave her."[12] Along with this, they mentioned the gymnastic costume frequently ("the style is graceful, and is becoming to almost everyone").[13] They liked its efficiency, and one of the movement's leaders, Frances Russell, even went so far as to suggest that it would be well accepted if, by some miracle, every college girl would appear in the streets wearing it in a modified form:

> Just imagine the college girls and society belles, who are *already* emancipated from the long drapery and corsets for the "business" of "physical culture," simply *extending the occasions upon which a comfortable and convenient costume may be worn.* The high-school girls would follow the college girls, and the clerks, typewriters, and all working girls would be with them; and you and I, with gray in our hair, would soon join in the glad procession, little girls of all sizes skipping in freedom by our sides.[14]

As we will see in Part Two, those college girls had the inclination to lead the way, but, initially at least, were held in check by their teachers, who represented an older generation and society at large. Clearly, Frances Russell understood the theory of fashion diffusion, but she misread her times. She would have to wait another generation for that diffusion to happen. But happen it did, and the gymnasium was the venue of success.

The dress reformers recommended the gymnasium dress for the housewife as well, with the suggestion that it would "materially lighten her labor." They made it clear, however, that she was to wear it only in private. Alice Stone Blackwell offered a neat compromise: "If it were necessary to go to the door, a long apron, which could be slipped on in a moment, would hide all peculiarities." Her comment reveals how deeply ingrained customary dress was even for these struggling women. Once again, we see that they argued vehemently for reform but remained timid in the application of it. Even their language betrays them. Blackwell hoped "that men, seeing their wives wearing a gymnastic dress during their working hours, would get accustomed to the costume, and would no longer be struck by it as something hideous and *outré.*[15] "Popular out-of-door sports and pastimes" provided another "potent aid" for their cause, according to the reformers:

> The seaside and mountain resorts have aided wonderfully in breaking
> the spell of conventionalism. Then the great and growing popularity
> of the bicycle with women is another factor not to be overlooked . . .
> even the universally loved and respected president of the Women's
> Christian Temperence Union chose a safety bicycle in preference to
> an outing at a resort distant from her charming home. The one draw-
> back to women's ease and comfort on the wheel is the long skirt. The
> bicycle is one of the many agencies acting for reform.[16]

At the end of 1893, the second symposium on the rational dress movement was held in conjunction with the Columbian Exposition, to assess the impact of the reformers' dress at the Chicago World's Fair, held during the six months from May through October.[17] Although the fair was a resounding triumph, reform dress was not. Visitors had demanded patterns for the reform dress (by now referred to as rational dress), which was basically a walking suit in all its fashionable guises, but without corsetry or long sweeping skirts. Above-the-ankle skirts with gaiters, and the divided skirt along the same lines as the gymnasium dress, were the alternatives to the fashion skirt. Patterns for looser bodices, often bloused, had appeared in *The Delineator* as yachting, tennis, and "outdoor sports" costumes as early as 1889, but these still called for a full-length skirt to complete the outfit.[18] The next year, however, versions of a new style introduced for "pedestrian and other athletic sports" featured skirts, shortened to low calf, that hid "Knickerbocker drawers" beneath them.[19] A separate pattern for knickerbockers, to be made, *The Delineator* suggested, out of wash silk, appeared in the same issue, with the recommendation that the garment be used for "traveling and outing uses."[20] Although these new styles for recreational activities seem, to our eyes, to answer the need of the dress reformers, the fair-goers complained that no patterns for rational dress were available to them. Eventually, Butterick introduced a pattern for the gymnasium bottom in response to the demand, but not in time for the fair. In fact, the complete patterns for bloomer costumes, including a variety of trousers, jackets

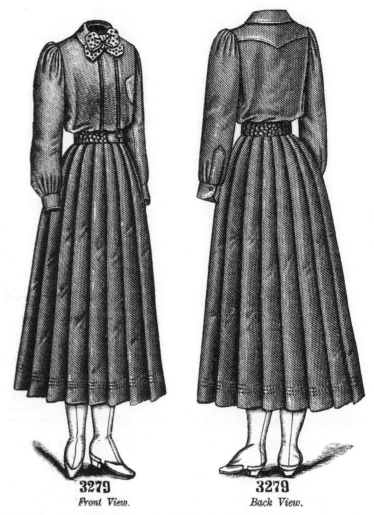

3279
Front View.

3279
Back View.

"Ladies' Costume. (Desirable for Pedestrianism)." Below the skirt, the legs are covered by gaiters. *The Delineator*, September 1891, 189.

and hats, did not appear in *The Delineator* until November 1894.[21] "Many women and men went home from the Fair disappointed because they saw not a single woman dressed in the new styles."[22] Chicago summers can be sweltering, so the demure and natty gaiters proved too hot, as did the sensibly firm fabrics used for the outfits. Besides that the clothes had no pockets. The leaders of the National Council of Women wore the reform dress only

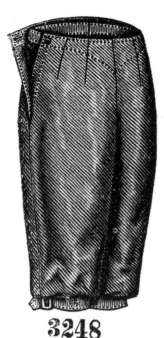

"Ladies' Knickerbocker Drawers. (Desirable for Travelling and Outing Uses)"—as long as they remained hidden under a skirt. *The Delineator*, May 1890, 363.

3248

occasionally, shrugging off their dismissal of it by saying, "In this latter day campaign, no one is asked to make a martyr of herself."[23]

Despite the leaders' reluctance to wear the sensible but offending garments, a photograph of "Mrs. Marie Reidesdelle in Her Bicycle Costume" was included in *The Arena*'s report on the symposium, which claimed, "This costume won the prize recently offered by the New York *Herald* for the best bicycle costume for ladies."[24] For this, Mrs. Reidesdelle won $50 (close to $1,000 in today's money) which surely must have eased any discomfort in wearing it. It consisted of "a divided skirt of two breadths of black cashmere (forty-eight inch goods, one breadth in each division), with tan leather gaiters meeting the divisions half way from the knee to the ankle." (No wonder women were reluctant to wear similar outfits in Chicago in the summertime.) Echoing other voices at other times, the article continued, "It seems a pity that this young woman, riding her wheel, to her business in this costume, feels obliged, because of its oddity, when off the wheel to cover it with a long skirt."[25]

Here, finally, we see the intersection of the dress reform movement with sport and outdoor activity. The report underscores the argument that, even

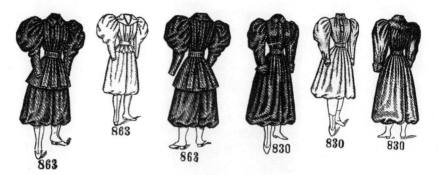

"Ladies' Bloomer Costume," patterns for reform dress, *The Delineator*, November 1894.

in the face of reform, dress worn in private could be functional, while dress worn in public had to conform to societal standards. And, as we have seen, although these standards were often influenced by the presence of men, women too carried high the banner of traditional dress.

How did the conservatism of high fashion greet the new craze of bicycling, which, by its very nature, epitomized a serious departure from the protected and demure expectations of the past? In a word, it adopted rational dress.

Fashion historiography rarely fails to mention the phenomenon of the bicycle and its influence in bringing about change in women's dress. But as we have seen, many other activities and trends also played significant roles. What bicycling brought to it was visibility. Repeatedly, as in the *New York Herald* article, contemporary American sources reinforced the notion that the bloomer or knickerbocker suit, almost invariably touted by later writers as bicycling garb, was not acceptable off the bicycle without a modest covering skirt, thereby negating much of the effect, and the effectiveness, of trousers.

Although the clothing was problematic, bicycling itself was a craze that engulfed not only the United States but the rest of the world as well. In the United States it exploded from some "100,000 wheelmen and women" in 1887 to universal acceptance by the time the fad ended around 1903. The bicycle became "the people's carriage," the "crowning luxury of the common people and the necessity of the well-to-do," including "the artisan, the millionaire, the professional man, the laborer, the rich merchant, the lady whose name appears in all the 'society movements of the day,' the shopgirl, the banker and his clerk." It was the "destroyer of caste and the annihilator of age."[26] In the three years that marked the height of the craze, 1895 through 1897, *Harper's Bazar* scattered comments, notices, and articles throughout its issues, offering readers all sorts of interesting tidbits about bicycling, including who was the latest to take up the fad. It turns out that everybody was— from aging women's rights advocates and female clergy to well-situated foreigners, stage stars, even royalty:"Miss Frances Willard's example in learning to ride the bicycle bids fair to be imitated by many other women of mature years. The Rev. Phebe A. Hanaford, who has left her first youth some distance behind her, is practising with the wheel"; "Madame Hanna Korany, of Syria, has become so far infected with Occidental ideas that she, too, is taking bicycle lessons."[27] Popular entertainers jumped on the bandwagon: "Bicycles have appeared upon the stage in variety shows and in exhibitions of fancy riding, but it has been reserved for M. Coquelin the younger to arrange a monologue to be recited from end to end as he wheels about the stage. He makes his entrance and his exit upon a 'machine' and varies his recitation by ringing his bell, blowing his whistle, and other appropriate 'business'"; "A curious but very pretty sight was the costume ride at the Michaux Cycle Club, Tuesday evening. Oddly enough, the bizarre costumes seemed particularly suitable to the wheel, and when the Virginia reel was danced (on bicycles) the effect was exceedingly good."[28] Not to be outdone, in an activity that should resonate with twenty-first-century readers, "Queen Margherita of Italy has added bicycle riding to mountain-climbing and the other active pursuits to which she has resorted in her endeavors to reduce her flesh. In this last form of exercise, as in the others, her example is imitated by the ladies of her court, no matter what their figures may be."[29] And in their coverage of the marriage of Princess Maud of Wales, daughter of the Prince of Wales and granddaughter to Queen Victoria, *Harper's Bazar* concluded, "She is a good shot, a fine wheelwoman, a capital amateur photographer, and an excellent performer on the violin."[30] The only wedding gift singled out for mention "was a band of white leather studded with turquoise. Six little bells of silver and gold, alternately, were strung on the band, which is attached to the handle bar of a bicycle."[31] As the magazine pointed out somewhat superfluously in October 1896, "bicycling is confined to no one class in England. Princess Victoria of Wales, Princess Charles of Denmark, and the Duchess of Connaught all ride wheels, and Lady Henry Somerset is said to be an enthusiastic cyclist."[32] Even an astonishingly nimble elderly rider was singled out for attention: "Probably the oldest woman who habitually rides a wheel is Miss Christina E. Yates, of Oakland, California. She is eighty years old, and although she has learned to ride within a year or so, she already has such skill that her teacher declares he means to instruct her in trick riding. She mounts her wheel every day, does not mind rough roads, and can cover a long distance without fatigue."[33]

More than one article reported on the denizens of Newport—"in that part of Newport, it goes without saying, in which fashions are stamped for the rest of the country." But Newporters, it seems, were slow in adopting the craze—until, that is, they saw that if it was good enough for foreign capitals, it must be good enough for Newport. Even the pronunciation changed, from the standard "bisick-ling" (or, to *Harper's Bazar*, "bicyc-ling") to "bicy-cling" (with a long *y* sound). "With this distinction, and this distinction alone," the magazine reported, "Newport consented to adopt it." Here, *Harper's Bazar* unwraps its sharpest critical needle, usually kept well hidden from its middle-class readership:

> "Bicyc-ling" was to be to the world outside just what it had always been—a convenient means of transportation, a cheap pastime, a wholesome exercise. With those who adopted "bicy-cling" such points of view were ignored. Indeed, they were never possible. Convenience, cheapness, and wholesomeness in Newport! Away with such things! What had they to do with "bicy-cling"? What had they, forsooth, to do with pleasure at all? As well discuss such subjects in relation to functions to be given in their palaces. One only vulgarized the whole affair. The privilege of a favored few is to enjoy the things for themselves.

(Interesting that foreign royalty was never criticized in these terms, only the American rich.)

But how Newport embraced the fad once they did!

> Everywhere in Newport, then, and on the roads outside, well-known people may now be seen on the wheel—young girls, middle-aged women, old men and boys, and those well-groomed young fellows who always bear about them unmistakable evidence, though subtle, of the well-to-do world to which they belong. Chaperons are not always

insisted upon. Greater liberty is allowed in going about on the bicycle than at any other time.[34]

Shades of the croquet craze before it! Newport had finally caught on.

Granted this reportage all came from a woman's magazine, but it is interesting to note that few men are mentioned in this list. Although men most decidedly rode, too, the phenomenon of cycling, certainly in these years of fashionability, seemed to belong more to women. And the magazine's readers were clearly avid for news about their favorite celebrities enjoying their favorite pastime.

There is no question that the bicycle gave women greater freedom than they had ever had before. Previously they had been limited to getting around in private carriages or on horseback, or if they could not afford those luxuries, public transportation and cabs, available only in cities. As a last resort, they depended on their own two feet. Now they were able to range about at will. A further advantage was that, by the time the craze hit, other sports-related activities had been well accepted into the mainstream of American life, so the appearance of women "wheeling" was less a cause for reproach than it might have been otherwise. In fact, as the bicycling craze passed its peak, another—golf—took its place, and the bicycle provided the means for golfers to get to the links. "So popular has golf grown," observed *Harper's Bazar* in 1897, "that it has actually caused bicycling to suffer a little in many places. Wheels are used, to be sure, but not so much for the purpose of taking long trips as for a means of getting to and from the golf course. . . . However, there is no need for cycling enthusiasts to worry. Theirs is, after all, the sport of the people *par excellence*, and can be enjoyed in hundreds of places where golf would be impracticable, and by thousands of persons who cannot spare the time or money for golf."[35] At that point, then, bicycling was becoming an accepted means of transportation.

So much has been written about the development of the bicycle and its evolution from a primitive two-wheel riding toy at the beginning of the nineteenth century to the safety bicycle of the late 1880s that there is no point in retelling that story in detail here.[36] Suffice it to say that the modern bicycle was made possible by two innovations: Charles Goodyear's vulcanization of rubber in 1839 (patented in 1844) and John Boyd Dunlop's invention of the pneumatic tire in 1888, which smoothed out the jarring and bumpy ride that enthusiasts had had to endure in the past.[37] By 1892, pneumatics had begun to take over the market.[38] Simultaneously with the appearance of the new tire came the safety frame, designed with two wheels of equal size and a reinforcing crossbar, which was "dropped" for women, creating the dropped-frame bicycle that accommodated their skirts.

Although it began life as a rather high-priced item, the safety bicycle was instantly embraced by the middle class. By 1896, Waverley was advertising its high-end bicycles ("America's Favorites" . . . built in the Largest and Best Equipped Factory on Earth") for $85 ("a clear saving of $15.00 or more"). At today's equivalent of close to $1,750, the bicycle did indeed represent an investment, especially when tire ads admitted that the best tires (the only ones "you are sure of getting home on if punctured") were "expensive"—but after all, they were the ones that made "the high-grade wheel."[39] Not all bicycles were that costly, of course. Another manufacturer offered a much wider range and advertised "high grade" bicycles at a discount if ordered by and shipped directly to the customer. A bicycle listed for $100 was reduced to $62.50; one for $85, to $45; $65 to $37.50; and $20 to $10. From these, you could choose either wood or steel rims, the wood being more expensive.[40] Another, Crescent Bicycles, offered bicycles ranging from $40 to $75, giving special attention to ladies with a "22 lb . . . . wheel . . . fitted with small rubber pedals, saddle specially designed for Ladies' use, up-curved handle bars, and high frame. It is, without doubt, the daintiest Ladies' Wheel on the market."[41] Yet another ad offered bicycles for as little as $10. Ads for and articles about bicycles appeared everywhere, in popular magazines, medical journals, cycling and outing weeklies and monthlies, even (and somewhat surprisingly) in the magazines strictly for women, such as *Harper's Bazar* and the fashion-oriented *Delineator*, whose main function was to display the newest styles and dress patterns available from Butterick. Indeed, on one page of the February 29, 1896, issue of *Harper's Bazar*, five out of six ads were for bicycles, further evidence of just how fashionable bicycling was during the mid-1890s.

In fact, bicycling, for a while at least, even eclipsed horseback riding. One article declared: "Cycling is far cheaper than horseback exercise, and throughout the last year or two this consideration has had its weight with many who never before thought of economizing in their sports. Its novelty, too, particularly in the case of women, has been in its favor, for a number who own saddle-horses have taken up wheeling, inspired perhaps by a desire for a change or by a spirit of investigation to see what the new sport is like."[42] (Note how issues of class insinuate themselves into the language of the women's magazines, even—or especially—on the subject of sports. As we saw with croquet and tennis, that was part of the appeal. And it is equally interesting to realize that average Americans had a tendency to defuse any hint of elitism by embracing each new sport as it came along.)

Cycling even lent a new look to horseback riding. *Harper's Bazar* columnist Adelia K. Brainerd commented one July, presumably during the midsummer heat, "I have observed two or three women riding [horses] in shirt-waists and straw sailor hats in the Park, instead of the conventional habit bodice and Derby or silk hat."[43] These hats and cotton waists, of course, presumably worn with standard riding skirts, were part of the uniform of the New Woman of the 1890s, and a much adopted style for the new bicyclists as well.[44] No doubt, though, even in the summer heat, women wore their customary corsets underneath. Indeed, the question of clothing in general for bicycling, and corsets in particular, occupied a great deal of print space, with fashion mavens, doctors, and sportsmen and sportswomen alike weighing in. But corsets (with some modifications) remained a constant. Generally then, the clothing for the sport was that of the fashionable 1890s, with the additional fillip of the dashing and daring rational dress thrown in, to the delight of onlookers and magazine writers alike. In the words of *Demorest's Family Magazine* in 1896, clothing for cycling was "a much discussed question."[45]

One result of the dress reformers' work, and an alternative to the ever-present corset, was what was known as the "health waist." This was a firm, sturdy underbodice cut to the natural waist without steels of any kind, but which gave what was believed to be much-needed support to the back.[46] It was designed with shoulder straps (rather like a tank top today), and could have reinforced seaming, or even lightweight boning, but broke from the strapless and tightly shaping tradition of the corset proper. It bound the torso, but not as rigidly as the shaped corset, which could be laced tightly, or not, as the wearer desired. In fact, in an era when even doctors regarded the (looser-laced) corseted body as the ideal female form, this garment really did represent a reform of sorts. So strong was the several-hundred-year tradition of corsetry that to leave them aside entirely was to label a woman

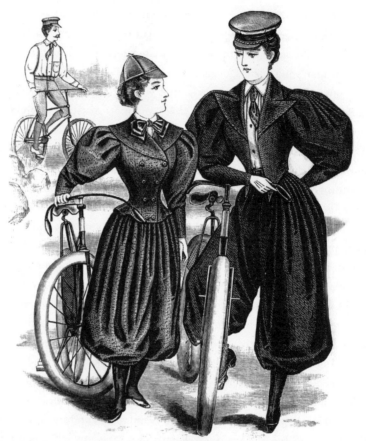

"Bicycling Outfits" from *The Delineator* leave no doubt that corsets were required even in summer to give the proper silhouette. Here, a girl and a woman are warmly covered in the fashionable balloon-sleeved jackets and Syrian divided skirt, whereas the man in the background wears only trousers and a shirt. *The Delineator*, August 1894, 168.

"loose." No self-respecting woman, certainly not the ones to whom the magazines directed their attention, would be caught without them. But they drew comment when worn on the bicycle. "Heavily boned waists are more comfortable than corsets to ride in," commented *Harper's Bazar*, "but for those who do not choose to discard the latter, there are now special designs, made shorter and more flexible than those for ordinary use."[47]

Kirk Munroe, identified as the "Founder of the League of American Wheelmen," challenged corset wearers in his article, "About Bicycles," which appeared in *The Book of Athletics and Out-of-Door Sports* in 1895:

As for the girl bicycle riders who, as a rule, put boys to shame by riding as straight as though they were on horseback, I am afraid that in
some cases they only do so because they can't bend over and breathe at
the same time. How is it, girls? Are not some of you trying to ride in
corsets, or at least tight waists [i.e., bodices] and belts? If so, you are
preparing yourselves a future of even greater suffering and unhappi-
ness than the monkey-like boys who bend low over their handlebars;
and to you, too, I would say that it were better never to have seen a
bicycle than attempt to ride under such conditions. Can you, when
dressed for a ride, raise your arms straight above your head and bring
the palms of your hands together? Can you stoop over and touch your
toes with the tips of your fingers without bending the knees? If you
can, your riding costume is all right. If you cannot, it is all wrong.[48]

The next year, *Harper's Bazar* got into the discussion:

The necessity for having the waist-clothing comparatively loose while
riding has been mentioned by many writers on the subject, but a little
observation will show that it will bear frequent repetition. What
pleasure there can be in the exercise to one whose gown is so tight that
she has trouble in drawing a long breath it is hard to discover, but the
ways of some women are truly past finding out. That there are not so
many offenders of this kind among cyclists as among horseback riders
is a sign of the increased allowance of common-sense which seems to
have accompanied the newer sport. Heavily boned waists are more
comfortable than corsets to ride in, but for those who do not choose to
discard the latter, there are now special designs, made shorter and
more flexible than those for ordinary use.[49]

The corset question as it concerned the bicycle was never resolved. Indeed,
it would take another chapter of sports history entirely to bring about
change in that quarter, as we will see in Part Two.

If the corset caused controversy, then the bloomer provoked dismay.[50] Early
on, women had found that long skirts and bicycle spokes were incompatible

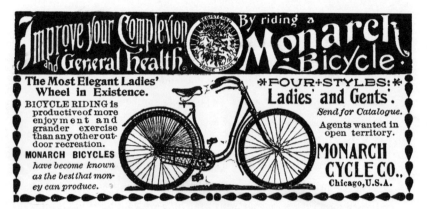

Advertisement for a Monarch drop-frame women's bicycle, complete with back wheel skirt guard, touting its healthful benefits. *The Delineator*, Columbian Number, May 1893, xxv.

for safe riding. The dangers of combining the two provided much fodder for commentary. But the fact remained: only two things could be modified, the clothing worn to ride and the bicycle itself. Some women chose the bloomer in one form or another, but many did not. For women who stuck to skirts, a number of possibilities presented themselves, none of them entirely satisfactory. The most notable one, and perhaps the overall favorite, was to modify the bicycle with the addition of a wire cage called a skirt guard. This encased the upper half of the rear wheel to prevent skirts from flapping back and tangling in spokes and chains. Of course, this added weight to the bicycle, which made it harder to manipulate or push when necessary, and prevented easy cleaning of the bicycle chain. Possibly in response to this problem, throughout the mid-1890s manufacturers tried to perfect a chainless gear system. Sometimes women removed either the rear-wheel mudguard or the chain guard (or both) to lessen the weight. "It seems to me that any woman who wears skirts when bicycling is reckless in removing her chain-guard," warned *Harper's Bazar's* "Out Door Woman." "Although one may ride for many miles and not happen to meet with an accident under these circumstances, there is always the danger of the skirts becoming entangled in some way, and when this occurs it almost invariably means a nasty fall." This suggested another solution, but one almost simultaneously dismissed because of fashion trends: "With an extremely short skirt [to the lower calf] there might be no possibility of trouble, but the recent tendency has been towards longer skirts." [51]

That comment was made in 1897, as the cycling craze was beginning to wane. But in the years immediately preceding, several kinds of skirts had been created for bicycling. The first was simply a shorter skirt, also used for and known as a "rainy day skirt."[52] This "short" skirt was some four to six inches shorter than the usual length. In its most extreme version, it could hit mid-calf. For the bicycling skirt, a favorite device was an opening that buttoned down the left side, or else box pleats falling from a yoke. Another version had a standard gored skirt front with a split pleat in the back (thereby making it a divided skirt), enabling the wearer to straddle the rear wheel. But by far the model most written about was the bicycle skirt that covered a pair of bloomers underneath. In November 1895 *The Delineator* published three pages of "Bicycle Garments" (all illustrated), offering readers some fifty Butterick patterns. Indeed, one wonders if the peak of the bicycling craze that began that same year was a direct result of these paper patterns, which offered cheap versions of the correct clothing to virtually any woman who could sew and could afford a bike and the cloth.

Here, everything a young girl or woman could ask for to look natty while on the wheel was at her fingertips, from full bloomer-bottomed (skirtless or skirted) bloomer suits to short skirts, jackets (Eton, Norfolk, and basque), shirtwaists with the enormous sleeves of the mid-1890s, hats and caps, knickerbockers, leggings, and gaiters.[53] The only thing missing was the health waist. *The Delineator* was very careful in its labeling to spell out the uses for each garment. The suits, or "Bloomer Costumes," offered a variety of choices: full bloomers, leaner Turkish trousers, or baggier Syrian divided skirts with fitted drawers to wear underneath. In fact, since the bloomers often called for accompanying underdrawers, a pattern for "Ladies' Knickerbocker Drawers" was offered as well. One skirt revealed that clever device so beloved by riders, "Ladies' Divided Cycling Skirt, having as Added Front-Gore and Plaits at the Back to Give the Effect of a Round Skirt when Standing," an all-important effect even when the "skirt" was a pair of trousers.[54] The following spring, Onlex advertised a cycling costume sold through New York's Best & Co. And lest potential buyers remain in any doubt, the wordy advertisement assured them of the efficacy of this superior garment, "made with a gored skirt in front and divided in the back, but in such a manner that it has the appearance of an ordinary skirt, the division not being perceptible either on the wheel or when used as an ordinary

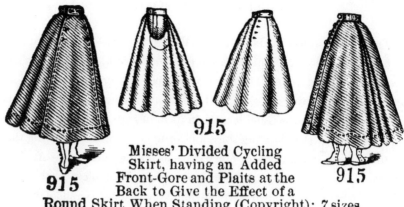

915

915

Misses' Divided Cycling Skirt, having an Added Front-Gore and Plaits at the Back to Give the Effect of a Round Skirt When Standing (Copyright): 7 sizes. Ages, 10 to 16 years. Any size, 1s. or 25 cents.

915

"Misses' Divided Cycling Skirt, having an Added Front-Gore and Plaits at the Back to Give the Effect of a Round Skirt When Standing." *The Delineator*, November 1895, iv.

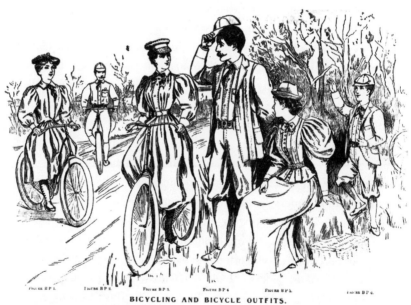

BICYCLING AND BICYCLE OUTFITS.

"Bicycling and Bicycle Outfits": "It is not a simple matter to effect abrupt and radical changes in customs that have prevailed for ages, and many women cyclists, therefore, cling to the essentially feminine skirt. . . . Those who adopt reforms readily have welcomed the new bloomers or trousers as a most radical innovation, and so rapidly has this fashion grown in favor that the so-called 'rational dress' is now worn without provoking comment." Comment, despite *The Delineator*'s enthusiastic claim, prevailed. *The Delineator*, April 1895, 579.

walking costume; at the same time it has all the advantages of a full divided skirt. It also has bloomers attached, which are not visible—is stylish, graceful and absolutely safe." Not to be outdone, on the very same page Best's rival B. Altman advertised a "Cycling Habit" (note the elite, horsey overtones), "The Improved Roycelle." Deemed ideal for wheeling, it offered "an ingenious arrangement of the drapery [that] combines many advantages of style, utility, and freedom of motion with a graceful and genteel appearance."[55] As the magazines had reported, every level of society embraced bicycling, and the ads quickly set out to find the high-end market.

Newport, of course, once it had accepted the new fad, had the advantage of being able to sport both singularly appropriate and more lavish and fragile, if inappropriate, clothes. *Harper's Bazar* left no doubt which it preferred:

> The best dressed women wear leggings and short skirts. Now and then one is seen in high-heeled slippers and silk stockings; but this is seldom, and only when the foot is very pretty and the thin stockings of a new design. And the young girl declares that they all dress this way in Paris without exciting comment, and that Newport is only a provincial old town for questioning the matter at all.
>
> The shirt-waist is all supreme. Sometimes it is a plain conventional affair of wash material, starched at the neck and wrist. Sometimes it is a dainty affair of mull that looks as though one day's experience would end its existence. Sometimes, but rarely, it is of chiffon. For the most part common-sense and good taste, which includes an instinct for the appropriate, rule in the question of a dress for the bicycle, and shirt-waists of wash material prevail, as they often do nowadays on horseback too.[56]

An 1895 *Harper's Bazar* article, "Smart Bicycling Suits," fleshed out *The Delineator's* illustrations with suggestions for fabrics and in the process gave home sewers or little dressmakers some tips from the greats. Linen, either English or Holland, was suitable for hot days, and tweed, serge, or even mohair for "uncertain" weather. "The choicest suits sent to Newport, Lenox, and Bar Harbor"—all the elite East Coast summer watering holes—"have a short skirt reaching to the shoe-top, covering knickerbockers buttoned or buckled just below the knee." Redfern, the famous London couturier (who by this time had expanded into both Paris and New York) known for his exquisite tailoring, and who gained his reputation as a tailor of women's riding habits, preferred "a kilt skirt with a broad box-pleat in front in genuine Highland fashion." In fact, Redfern had made two suits for each of the six American women in a company of twelve cyclists who were heading off to England and France that summer, taking their wheels with them. Many skirts opened down the left side, said the magazine, but "tailors consider it better to button them half-way down each side of the skirt front, as they are then very easily dropped." Skirts were lined throughout, but had no stiffening. Knickerbockers were narrower, even though they took the place of all petticoats. The best ones were sewn to a hip yoke to smooth the line under the skirt. In the summer, silk pongee was recommended for the knickerbockers; those made out of a rough Scotch wool for cooler weather were to be lined, preferably with silk serge or cotton sateen. The bloomers were "short," but the skirts reached the ankle. Gaiters completed the look.[57]

As for the jackets, in that year of the fullest sleeves ever, they had to have sleeves that were "ample enough to go on over those of a shirt-waist without crushing them," a thankless if not impossible task. As for the shirtwaists themselves, those of "cotton or of wash silk are precisely like those in use for other suits, each cyclist knowing what best becomes her." The preferred colors were drab so that dust would not show, but *Harper's Bazar* also recommended brown, black, and navy, often with a white or cream contrast. Lastly, "summer gloves for bicyclists are of finely woven lisle thread, with the inner side of the palm and fingers covered with heavy kid. They are fastened by four buttons, are worn very large, and cost $1.25 a pair."[58]

The following year's June 13 issue of *Harper's Bazar* provided a wealth of information about the cost of a complete outfit for the well-dressed cyclist. Ever attuned to its reading public, the magazine offered alternatives, going first for high quality, then for moderate. "Bicycling is to be more the fashion than ever at the watering-places," it reported, "and at least two bicycle costumes must needs be provided for summer wear—one of serge, cheviot, or covert-cloth for cool days, and one of linen, Russian crash, or the wiry material that looks like hair-cloth, or perhaps white duck for the hot weather." Much discussion regarding various styles followed, culminating in the anointing of the preferred one: "The Eton jacket is the most useful, on account of being so light and small that it can be carried on the handle-bar if it is not desired to wear it." Even so, the writer noted that it had to be cut long enough in the back to cover the belt of the skirt. Heaven forfend the waistband should show. Generally, "the tailors prefer the double-faced cloth for their heavy costumes" since it hangs better. But this cloth "is always expensive," and a "handsome costume" made from it would cost in the neighborhood of $50. Of course, this included the waist or coat lined with silk. When we realize that $50 would equal $1,020 in today's dollars (plus another $25 for the gloves), we can see that this indeed would be a very expensive outfit to wear for bicyling, and far out of reach of the average middle-class budget. Linen, it seemed, offered a better choice. "In the linens there are some marvellous fabrics. One that looks like covert cloth is only 15 cents a yard, makes up very well, and launders well. A costume just made of this material, recently finished, only costs $7, including all the findings. It was made by a cheap dressmaker, to be sure, who copied the model in one of the newest patterns." Although $7 looks much more affordable, it still amounts to some $145 in today's dollars. But several of the New York stores were advertising suits that June for as little as $5. Some were eminently suitable for cycling, with only a little adjustment here and there—taking a breadth out of the skirt back, for example, to make it narrower—and at an equivalent cost of just over $100 (on sale), it begins to look like a middle-class outfit after all. Of course, the wearer would have to use her own "inevitable shirt-waist" and decide what she should wear underneath. Pongee silk and colored lawn were good, but "Lansdowne or gloria silk" were "very wide, exceedingly cool, and only cost a dollar a yard." Of course, that is still close to $20 per yard in our terms. Clothing was clearly not inexpensive in the nineteenth century, even when a woman made it herself or hired a "cheap" dressmaker.[59] Not until the twentieth century, with the invention of manufactured fibers and clothing designed to fit more loosely, thereby permitting mass manufacturing, did the cost of clothes drop.

One thing is apparent from all these articles: bloomers were a highly recommended part of the bicycling gear for women. But equally apparent is the understanding that they were absolutely not to show, especially off the wheel. Recall Marie Reidesdelle's prizewinning costume from 1893, designed on the Syrian trouser model and worn with boots and gaiters. Even as the newspaper reporter admired it for its attractiveness and efficiency, he was bemused by the fact that she had to cover it with a skirt while not riding.

The popular press kept the news of the bicycle bloomer alive for its readers. Letters in the Wellesley College Archives, however, tell us perhaps more clearly than anything else just what it must have been like for the young woman of that day to experience the new world of bicycling and the new kinds of clothing she needed for it. Louise N. Pierce entered Wellesley in September 1896. In October, she wrote a long letter home to her mother, bringing her family in Maine up to date on what she was doing at school—or, more precisely, what she was wearing or wanted to be able to wear. She had recently bought a hat, "just like a man's except that there is a cock's feather in it. If I don't like it Papa can have it. I think I shall get a cap. Most all the girls wear one. My hat is soft felt, dark brown, cost two and a half." She mentions that she has also bought a pair of gaiters, which, as we have seen, were so often included in outfits for bicycling to cover the shins. Hers were the "jersey kind." They "come above the knee, cost a dollar and a half."[60] Then, after mulling over what she needed for winter wear, she declared:

> If I come back another year I want a new bicycle. Everybody rides here, and I don't wonder the roads are simply fine. It's quite flat around, and the streets are broad and smooth, not stony at all, a good deal like asphalt. It's the best place I ever struck for wheeling.[61] Yesterday Dora and I hired wheels and together with Miss Yeater and Harriet Righter went riding. Had an awfully good time. Staid an hour and a half. Cost thirty cents. I wore my short skirt, bloomers and gaiters. I never rode in a regulation suit before. They're great. Shant ever ride in any other kind. The skirt is all right, it's pretty short, it seems very short to me; if I don't like it I can have it changed at Xmas. The blouse is OK.

Louise's letters, like so many written home to their parents, tell us a great deal about the lives of the college girls, including a surprising amount about their clothing.[62] Earlier that same October, Louise had written to her mother about a rainy day skirt. What is interesting here is that it was her mother who had suggested the new style; Louise was reluctant to adopt it. Perhaps, to judge by her comment about the short cycling skirt, she was uncomfortable wearing the new length. But peer pressure had done wonders. (Probably her mother had whipped up the skirt and its bloomers and matching blouse and sent them off to her daughter for her comment. Where else would the new bicycle suit have come from?) Louise wrote:

> A good many of the girls here wear short skirts on rainy days, like you wanted to make me, and if you have time, you might want to make me one. Some have them come to above their shoe tops, but I think *to* the tops is short enough. I have measured as well as I can and think it made, but without binding would be about 31 inches. That's 5 in. shorter than this black everyday skirt and make some long gaiters too. Tell me how to measure for them. I think the serge would be better than the broadcloth, even if the bloomers are of that for it isn't so heavy and won't catch the dirt so badly, I don't believe, for I've just been comparing mine with Lena's. And the serge matches the sweater better. They make them with about 6 in. of stiffening around the bottom to keep it down. I can use it for a bicycle skirt when I ride again. about as wide as my usual skirts Lined perhaps with rustle cambric.

At least among Wellesley girls, the bicycle suit seems to have been a hit.[63] One would expect that if it were to be accepted anywhere, it would be on college campuses. As for the rest of the world, it is hard to assess just how widespread the use of the bloomer or "divided skirt" actually was. From cartoons, drawings, and other views from popular sources of the time, it would appear that daring and dashing women wore them everywhere, to the amusement or consternation—and even the admiration, in a few rare cases—of onlookers, mostly men. Other sources suggest that if it caught on anywhere, it was in France, where it was worn by women members of cycling clubs who congregated in Paris's Bois de Boulogne. Hattie C. Flower, one of the dress reformers whose work was reported in *The Arena*, wrote in 1893, "The divided bicycle dress is so common in Paris as to excite no remark."[64] We saw earlier the Newport girl's shrugged comment about

Frenchwomen and their dress for cycling. Perhaps she was exaggerating, as American and English women frequently did when speaking of French women, in what would appear to be a mixture of admiration, scornful superiority, and envy. In fact, the truth about the French and the bicycle seems very little different from American and English women's experiences.

France, too, had responded to the bicycle with wild enthusiasm. Indeed, early versions of it had originated in France. As in the United States and England, the French also published magazines, books, and articles detailing every aspect of the joys of cycling. And certainly the bloomer costume appeared there as it had everywhere else. But in 1894 a leading French magazine, *La Bicyclette*, seemed ambivalent in its reaction to women cyclists. Although it used a drawing of a woman bicycling on its cover, it showed her wearing a sailor dress hiked to the knee—sporty, but definitely without bloomers.[65] In fact, very much as in the United States and Great Britain, a reference to the bloomer appeared in a poem making fun of a comely bloomer-clad skater. It was illustrated, again showing the garment hiked up above the knee. The poem ends: "[the skater,] feverishly sportive, . . . pursued her ill-considered course / without fear of what anyone would say."[66] An article in the same issue, however, "Nouvelles d'Angleterre" (News from England), reported on a meeting of the Ladies Cyclists Club there, where members discussed and "vigorously defended the new costume," which was being "so cruelly attacked by some distressed souls." The women were not intimidated by these attacks, indeed were "enchanted" to be able to wear the "culotte," did not want to give it up, and hoped to be able to wear it not only for sporting exercises but in their daily lives as well. "Whoa! Not so fast, if you please, ladies!" gasped the French magazine. That time had not yet come; the idea was embryonic at best, and "impossible at the moment."[67]

Later that month the same magazine ran an ad for cigarette papers (decidedly male-directed), using as its come-on a drawing of a woman on a bicycle holding a cigarette and wearing a bicycling outfit with a man-tailored jacket and shirt, but with a very tight (obviously corseted) waist, short, knee-length skirt, and narrow jodhpur-like trousers and boots underneath—saucy, racy, definitely pin-up material.[68] In February, H. Fraenkel, Paris, advertised "Costumes pour Vélocipédistes."[69] Both the man and woman in the ad are shown wearing men's tailored trousered suits, his a knickerbocker suit, hers a bloomer. And later that month, another illustration of a poem shows a woman leaning on a fence outside an empty house wearing a bloomer costume.[70] It seems, then, that images of women wearing the "new outfit" illustrated poems, stories, and ads to draw in the reader (usually male), but very few articles actually discussed women bicycling.

Perhaps more than anything else, a three-part serialized story in *La Bicyclette*, "Pourquoi Elles Pédalent, Une Conversation," carried on between twenty-three-year-old Suzanne and her husband, thirty-one-year-old Octave, reveals the view of women cyclists and the bloomer costume from both sides of the fence. From this tale, we realize that there really is not a great difference between French attitudes and anyone else's.[71] The story revolves around an ongoing argument between the two centering on Suzanne's bicycle riding with her friends. Octave doesn't like Suzanne's friends and her cycling, and as she leaves, dressed for the sport, the argument mounts. He insists that she go back into the house to change her clothes. She is outraged, but he is adamant, telling her that her outfit is ridiculous and indecent.

"Ridiculous! Indecent!" she gasps. "A costume that came from Redfern!"

"I don't care where it came from," he snorts. "It isn't any the less grotesque! You, Madame, you, a respectable woman, you promenade in trousers, in broad daylight, all over Paris! It's disgraceful!"

Essentially she answers that she wears it only in the Bois and isn't hurting anybody. Besides, all the fashionable women (that is, her friends) are doing it.

"Those creatures!" he scoffs. They and she are only coquettes on "stupid two-wheeled machines," making spectacles of themselves in the company of young idiots whose cavalier manners are repugnant.

As with any good argument, she counterattacks. While he says it is stupid for her to ride a bicycle, she says he is a beast for not even trying it. Her doctor has told her that fresh air and exercise are good for her health; he retorts that she is refusing to grow up. Is that so, she snaps. Just look at me in this costume. See how well it fits! Look how alluring I am in it! Not too alluring, he answers. But then she tells him how freeing cycling is, how good it feels, like flying, without fatigue, without fetters. "It's delicious!" Finally, he agrees to go with her, "but not today." And she must go for walks with him, and with him alone.

The second part of this little morality tale takes place in the shop of Suzanne's couturier, "M. Frédéric." When she consults him on a new costume for cycling, he answers that the matter is very delicate since cycling is "un sport de noblesse," too relatively recent for any rules to have been adopted. But she replies that he must devise some rules. Other sports, he says, have their own rules. Riding, for example. The woman mounts her horse, her habit adjusted exactly and, like the man's outfit, skin-tight. Her long gown covers her feet perfectly, giving aesthetic perfection.

But riding a bicycle is very different, she counters. The wind, the sun, the dust on this machine without any sides require a comfortable outfit.

"But, Madame," he demands. "How important is it, in the matter of feminine costume, to be comfortable? To be hygienic? Is it chic or isn't it chic? Everything boils down to that, says the Prince."

"Ah, the Prince." She had run into him "en bicyclette" along with a delicious young woman wearing "a costume" just the other day.

"Quick! Quick, a description of the costume of this woman!"

Goodness, she replies, they were going by so fast she hardly had time to notice. But, "Wait. I think she wore white cheviot, or very light, in any case, with a matching bolero and culotte bouffante [full bloomers] . . ."

"Stop, stop, Madame, make sure. *En culotte*, did you say?"

"Yes, yes. Bloomers, or at least a combination skirt of some sort, or something like that."

"Was she or was she not en culotte? That is the question, as the divine Shakespeare said. Skirt or bloomers. That is the problem whose solution will eternally single out the master of the art. What's your opinion on this, Madame?"

Their conversation continues.

"Well, it seems to me that bloomers are very becoming . . ."

"Evidently it's becoming, especially on you, with your charming figure. . . . The bloomer would be good-looking on any woman with a good figure. Is it worn well? Would a woman of the world hesitate to sport it in public?" He plunges into meditation.

"The skirt is so inconvenient . . . ," she says.

"Didn't I just tell you that convenience, comfort, and so on have nothing to do with feminine costume? Is it chic or isn't it chic?"

"Do you want me to go and ask the prince?"

"What an idea! Interview him adroitly. I won't make my judgment until I have his high appreciation. The question is too new."

And off she goes to check out the style with the prince.

The third and final episode returns to the married protagonists. They are now on vacation. Just before going to bed, they talk about going on a bicycle trip the next day. Octave mentions that he has allowed Suzanne to order a new bicycle costume from the couturière. (Notice the feminine form of the word. Clearly, it is not M. Frédéric.)

"Ah, speaking of the costume, it's very pretty!" she retorts sarcastically. "Thanks to you, I will have the air of a Quaker with my long skirt and my big coattails. . . . My couturière is a provincial. She knows nothing about chic." As we have learned above, there can be no greater condemnation.

All the French magazines seem to prove that the struggle women had in other countries took place in France as well. There is no question that the bloomer outfit (or the *costume en culotte*) was favored by the Suzannes of the cycling world, but probably there is no question either that their husbands thought very much as Octave did. (Indeed, his reactions remind us keenly of Pierre de Coubertin's at the time of the first Olympic Games. Both were men of their generation and place.) And there is also no doubt that the women's cycling clubs, elitist all, gathered in the Bois and cycled together there, wearing their bloomer outfits. But they were not welcome to do so anywhere else in the city. That is equally clear. In fact, most women seem to have worn some version of the bicycle skirt, perhaps with bloomers underneath.[72]

As in the United States, patterns became available for the home sewer or little dressmaker, tucked into the women's magazines on pull-out tissue. The *Journal de Demoiselles* included patterns for high-style Amazones, or riding habits, in 1891, 1892, and 1894, and bathing dress patterns in 1892, 1893, and 1894. In 1895 the magazine became the *Petit Courrier des Dames*. Not a word about bicycle outfits appeared until June 1895, when two costumes designed by Mme Gradoz were described, but without patterns. Both had bloomers. Another pair of outfits by the same designer, variations on the theme, appeared the next year. Finally, in October 1897, a complete tissue paper pattern for a cyclist's costume, including jacket, pantaloon, vest, and belt, appeared, but without any article describing it or any accompanying illustration other than the one on the pattern itself. By 1898, not a single word about sport or bicycling appeared during the entire twelve months of the magazine. Nothing could have indicated more clearly that the bicycle bubble had finally burst.

Overall, it is safe to say that Frenchwomen weren't regarded very seriously as bicyclists, and that in fact the Anglo-American belief that Frenchwomen could wear anything without criticism was simply not true. Almost as if in an attempt to codify the stereotype, France's own belittling press seemed to imply that Frenchwomen's only real interest was in the clothes, and in trying to figure out what to wear. As usual, women were made fun of in the process.

England too made fun of its women on bicycles. *Punch* had a field day, publishing cartoons and quips throughout the peak years of the craze, which of course lent the bloomer outfit a certain dubious notoriety. But at least one observer of the time reported in later years that the trousers "were hardly ever seen in reality."[73] Even Lady Harberton, that doughty leader of English dress reform, admitted in a letter written in 1899: "Quite between ourselves I am sure there are less wearing it than there were a year ago, and very many less than there were two years ago. . . . Except for myself I don't think I have seen one this winter!"[74] Most women wore a regular skirt, or if they did wear a bloomer, covered it with a skirt that they carried with them as they rode.

The reasons for this decline are not entirely clear. Perhaps the traditional need to wear skirts at all times, what I call the skirt convention, was too strong to buck. Perhaps the costs of such a narrowly dedicated outfit were prohibitive for most women. Perhaps women simply got tired of defending themselves from the onslaughts of the critics and the ridicule of the populace at large. Whatever the reasons, *Harper's Bazar* commented on the trend away from trousers as early as May 1896. In an "Outdoor Woman" column the magazine revealed a number of things: first, its awareness of the fashion process and the regionalism of fashion in the United States; second (as M. Frédéric had insisted to the feckless Suzanne), that practicality and comfort had nothing to do with fashion; and last, what may perhaps have been the most compelling reason of all:

> One of the first things which the opening of the cycling season has
> brought to light is a fact of much interest to the average woman: it is
> the decline and fall from favor of the bloomer. The question which

was pending during last season as to whether this costume was destined to succeed and eventually supercede all others has been practically settled—at least as far as New York and the East in general are concerned. Throughout the West the "radical dress," in all its varieties, is still very popular, and probably claims more adherents than it ever did here. Always fond of novelties, our Western sisters may be loathe to relinquish the garment, which undeniably has several good qualities to recommend it, but, judging from the Atlantic seaboard, the reaction which is now felt here will surely extend to them in time.

There is just one reason for the failure of the bloomers, but that one is all-sufficient. They are safe; they are comfortable; they are entirely modest, despite criticisms to the contrary; pretty and becoming most emphatically they are not, and this has been their death-blow. Occasionally, when exceptionally well cut, and worn by a pretty woman, with a trim, neatly proportioned figure, they were not unpleasing; but this conjunction of circumstances was rare.

To hammer home the point, the writer continued, "Women are too anxious about their personal appearance to be willing to wear what their own eyes tell them is ugly, and though it took a little time to discover it, this was the unfortunate adjective which nearly always applied to the bloomers." To reassure readers, the columnist lauded the new shorter skirts, even the divided skirt, which, if made "not too long," presented "no difficulties worth mentioning." Finally, the writer relegated the bloomer to its proper place: "It ought to be said, by-the-way, that while bloomers as an outside garment are not desirable, they are far and away the best things to wear under a skirt. Petticoats are only an embarrassing nuisance on a wheel."[75]

Ultimately, the impact of bicycling and its clothing was probably felt more elsewhere than while wheeling. *Harper's Bazar* claimed in 1897 that "the effect of the bicycle as expressed in the dress it introduced has had a widespread influence upon skating costumes this year. The short skirt is worn to a great extent, and has been taken up eagerly by the most expert skaters." It was safer, more convenient, and more suitable for skating than "ordinary length" skirts, which tended to become wet and "draggled around the bottom" and to get caught in the blades when the skater attempted fancy steps.[76] *The Ladies' World,* a Boston publication, bore this out in 1898 as it discussed what to wear for "rainy day dress":

> The first move, of course, which naturally suggests itself, is the short-ening of the skirt. So much freedom has been conceded to the bicycler in the matter of abbreviated skirts that the suggestion does not send a chill of horror over one's whole being as it otherwise would. So the women who are obliged to be out in all weathers owe much to the wheel, for it is a great comfort to be able to walk the streets in a com-fortable, short skirt and not be the cynosure of all eyes, both mascu-line and feminine. . . .
>
> Petticoats must be discarded, being superceded by warm woolen bloomers. Talk about the emancipated woman! The right to earn her own living on terms of equality with man, to vie with him in work, sport or politics, to vote, to hold office, to be president as well as queen and empress, would never bring the blessed sense of freedom that an outdoor costume, sans trailing skirts and entangling folds and plus a short skirt and bloomers, gives to the average woman. . . .
>
> Bear in mind that these articles [bloomers] are worn in place of the petticoat, *over* and not instead of the ordinary underwear, consist-ing of woven woolen drawers or union suit, and when the weather is severe, tights should be added, under the bloomers, of course.[77]

Boston was a center of dress reform—*The Arena* was published there—and certainly it was the major metropolitan center closest to many women's schools in the East. And yet, as late as 1898, this article appeared to instruct women on the correct way to manage the "new" garments. Most telling of all is the fact that, after the bicycling craze had completely passed some-time around 1903, pushed aside by the appearance of the automobile, so had the furor over the bloomer suit. It was not seen in public again. It retreated to the playing grounds and gymnasiums of the universities and colleges where it had come from in the first place.

Thus, though it has become much loved by costume historians for its sig-nificance, the cycling costume of bloomers and tailored top did not, in the long run, either last or greatly influence other dress. When the dust had cleared, the skirt convention had reasserted itself, even for bicycling. We get an eerie sense of déjà vu at this point when we realize that the fate of the bicycle bloomer was exactly the same as the fate of the Bloomer Costume worn for skating some thirty years before, in the 1860s. While women were out of doors in the company of men, they wore skirts.

The lasting influence for permanent change came instead from the field of women's education and the clothing worn for it. Bloomers continued to be worn in schools, but not for another twenty-plus years would women dare to go out in public wearing knickers, uncovered by demure skirts. Sports, then, embraced by both men and women alike and often played together, demanded a gradual easing of clothing, but certainly nothing outside the fashion impulses keeping step with them.

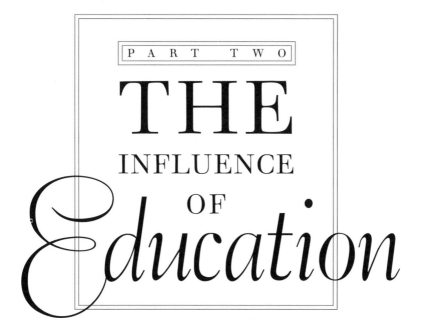

PART TWO

THE

INFLUENCE

OF

Education

PRIVATE CLOTHING
FOR
Physical Education

In Part One we saw the rise of various outdoor games, sports, and pastimes that became popular in the nineteenth century. The clothing that women wore for them was, as we have seen, simply the fashion of the day, suitable for mixed company. A few minor modifications allowed for the physical demands, if any, of the activities. If women got into trouble over the clothing they chose to wear, it was generally because they overstepped the limits of acceptability. Invariably, the difficulties arose when they wanted to wear trousers, as with the bicycle bloomer. Throughout the entire nineteenth century, men—and many women, too—had difficulty accepting women in pants and enjoyed ridiculing them. The reportage on women wearing the bloomer was peppered with almost as much rhetoric against them as for them, and certainly the most memorable images were the cartoons that laughed them to scorn.

In Part Two, then, we will look at the developments that helped women finally overcome that hurdle—developments that paralleled in time the rise of the sports and games discussed in Part One. It was a slow process. Most of the clothing that emerged, all based on Amelia Bloomer's costume, was hidden from view in private homes, in spas, even in the new gymnasiums that were being built. Ultimately, though, it found recognition within the confines of women's higher education, where for the first time women were encouraged to wear practical clothing for exercise in segregated educational communities, more or less away from men. This new type of trousered dress, designed to answer need, was the clothing of physical education. By its very nature, unlike the clothing for sport, it was private clothing, never meant to be seen in public. Subversion was probably the farthest thing from the minds of the women who instigated this new kind of dress, but subversive it was—and, as is often the case with subversion, it was ultimately successful as well.

The chapters that follow describe the second prong of our story, the development of the clothing that today we call sportswear. As we saw in Part One, which dealt with the public arena, the atmosphere of the time was ripe for change. Women were eager to be outdoors, to be active, to be doing. But the next part of the story provides the key. Without it, the sea change in women's dress in the early twentieth century could not have taken place. Acceptance of new ideas about clothing had to begin somewhere, and as we have seen, it certainly wasn't about to happen in the public sphere. If anything could have brought it about, it would have been the bicycle craze, embraced with such enthusiasm by all classes everywhere. Yet even its widespread popularity could not break down the rigid expectations and limitations in the matter of dress. It would take a completely different venue to bring that about—the venue of women's education.

Many of the same factors, trends, and people that helped to stimulate interest in sports also affected the thinking about women's education at the time. Indeed, many of the reformers worked in more than one arena. Here, then, we will meet again a number of the people to whom we have already been introduced. Rather than being strictly parallel, though, the two developments weave back and forth, touching from time to time. Finally, they came together as a whole in the middle years of the twentieth century.

One fact remains constant throughout both parts of the story: women of the nineteenth century lived in an atmosphere rigidly controlled by the separation of male and female roles and the attendant conventions that formed what has been called the cult of true womanhood. Every aspect of both men's and women's lives fell within this framework, and for the most part, all were happy to have it this way. It would be presumptuous of us as twenty-first-century observers to criticize this arrangement. It was simply the zeitgeist of the era.[1] But because of this separation, even in the privacy of women's institutions of higher education, certain niceties were observed. As Ellen W. Gerber delicately commented in The American Woman in Sport, *the physical education programs of the nineteenth century "required dress and activities that the women teachers thought were best performed in female seclusion." But performed they were, in spite of—or perhaps because of—women's knowledge that they would never be allowed this freedom "outside." A Vassar graduate remembered playing baseball at the college in the 1870s and recalled that "the public, so far as it knew of our playing, was shocked, but in our retired grounds, and protected from observation even in these grounds by sheltering trees, we continued to play in spite of a censorious public."[2]*

Not every school eliminated all men, of course; close family members, even "diplomatic cousins" were occasionally permitted. Lizzie Southgate Parker, in her essay "Physical Culture at Smith," written in 1890 or 1891, noted that "frequently during the class the platform of the gymnasium was filled with visitors, the masculine element being confined to fathers and uncles, with a very limited supply of cousins who might by extraordinary diplomacy secure admittance."[3] On the other hand, another alumna reminisced many years after the fact that all she remembered about a basketball game held among the Smith girls in the early 1900s was the crowd of Amherst boys in the balcony. But that was later; in the early days, men were forbidden entry altogether. This freed the Smith girls from the self-consciousness that they might feel playing in front of young men while wearing the strange clothing developed for sports—clothing designed not to be seen outside the gym.

Reference after reference throughout this entire period attests to the separation of private and public, the need to guard women from male view while doing exercise (and therefore wearing exercise clothes). In fact, some of the most ardent advocates of the Victorian ideals of true womanhood were the teachers of physical education themselves. They believed that a woman "should always preserve her inborn sense of modesty and innocence; she must never be seen by the opposite sex when she is likely to forget herself," meaning, as Gerber explained lest it be misinterpreted by later generations, that she was "caught in the emotional excite-

ment of an important contest."⁴ To aid in the adherence to such ideals, directors of physical education mandated that skirts must always be worn over gymnastic costumes when the girls walked to or from the playing fields or outdoor courts, or crossed public streets. This would hide their "irregular" gym clothes from public view. (Shades of the skirts worn over the bicycle bloomers.)⁵ No small matter, this, as we see from gymnastics teacher Gertrude Walker's plea in her "Report of the Department of Physical Culture in Smith College, From 1886 to 1888" at the alumnae meeting of June 19, 1888. After a list of requests, she added, "We ought also to have dressing-rooms furnished with lockers, so that the young ladies could dress and undress in the building and in this way escape from the exposure that so many are now obliged to risk in going to and from their boarding places." Whether she believed in her own argument or used it only because she understood her audience so well, we will never know. We do know, though, that her eloquence proved effective. The alumnae went to work raising funds for the new gymnasium, stung, no doubt, by the realization that their alma mater was "surpassed in ... facilities by Vassar, Bryn Mawr, and even some seminaries."⁶ They planned events ranging from "begging boldly," to selling commencement poems, to having Mark Twain read from his works at Smith.⁷ And they were successful: in 1890, the new gymnasium opened.⁸

Mount Holyoke College also required the cover-up skirt. As the unknown author of a "History of the Physical Education Department" remembered: "During this time [the turn of the century] skirts had to be worn over the bloomers whenever a student walked on campus. I believe this was a college policy but the physical education director [whose name was Lord] was blamed for it." The students even went so far as to compose a ditty that went, "Who is on the Lord's side, Who will wear a skirt? . . . For she's as mean as dirt."⁹ Clearly this was not a popular policy with the students, but it remained in effect nonetheless. At both Smith and Mount Holyoke, the only place the girls could wear their gym suits was in the gymnasium. As Lizzie Southgate Parker remembered, "These hours were thoroughly enjoyable when once we were in the gymnasium, but it was always an interruption to be obliged, in the middle of the afternoon, to array ourselves in the gymnasium costume . . . and to return to 'citizen's dress' before tea."¹⁰

To underscore just how seriously this separation for modesty's sake was taken, we turn to the most exciting event of the Smith school year, the basketball game between the sophomores and the freshmen. Although it was momentous enough to merit complete coverage in the Boston Globe, *it was an event for girls only. Senda Berenson, the basketball teacher, posted an unequivocal note on the gymnasium door, which can be found today in the college archives. It reads flatly, "Gentlemen are not allowed in the gymnasium during basketball games." To remove men was to remove a major source of self-consciousness. And to remove self-consciousness was to open up possibilities for creativity, growth, change, and freedom.*

The approach as we see it played out here was confined strictly to the gymnasium, but as it broadened to undergird the entire educational environment for women, it offered a whole new atmosphere, not simply in their activities and their clothing for it, but in their thinking, in their lives. The women's colleges particularly encouraged women's growth from the beginning. These schools were an intriguing, even daring mix of the traditional and the experimental, of the conventional and the extraordinary. But they made educated womanhood their goal, rather than merely being willing to add women, almost as an afterthought, to the schools already educating men.[11] Of course, the women's colleges remained firmly embedded within the Victorian realm of women's sphere; but even there, because of their self-imposed isolation, they were willing and able to experiment with new ideas, whether it was to do with curriculum—offering Latin and the classics as well as the new sciences such as zoology to women, unheard of elsewhere at the time—or exercise and new games. Nowhere else could women blossom so fully.

Because of this, change could finally take place.

TROUSER
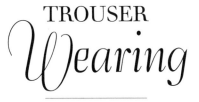
Wearing

Early Influences

TROUSER WEARING IN THE WEST WAS A JEALOUSLY GUARDED MALE prerogative and remained so for over five hundred years. Over the centuries, women adapted many styles and items of clothing from the men of their time, everything from doublets and ruffs, to Cavalier beaver hats, to redingotes and spencers, to starched collars, ties, boaters, and bowlers—even high heels. But the one thing they could not touch, it seemed, was any kind of bifurcated garment, or trousers. As we have seen, each time women appeared in public wearing them, they were ridiculed to such an extent that they just gave up, sensing, no doubt, that other more worthwhile battles could be fought—and won—elsewhere in the continuing war between the sexes. Why men felt the need to protect this sartorial right above all others is not entirely clear, especially when the history of pants is not particularly noble. Perhaps then, as now, men were leery of the power of women, and giving them this very visible equalizer might prove too dangerous in the delicate balance of the world. It is a question that may remain forever unanswered.

Trousers—ankle-length, straight-cut tubes that loosely encased each leg—were humble in origin, worn by male peasants and countrymen centuries before anyone else in the Western world thought of adopting them. Sailors began to wear them, probably in the seventeenth century, certainly in the eighteenth. Loose-fitting—covering the knee but not the ankle—and usually mass-produced out of cheap cloth, they became known as "slops."[1] Another surprising application, and one that may have had some influence if only because of its early appearance and ultimate longevity, was in the popular commedia dell'arte, in the costumes for Harlequin, Pierrot, and a number of other characters who were customarily dressed in straight pants.[2] Just as the actors portrayed stock characters reacting to stock situations, so too their stock costumes identified them to the audience. Several male performers wore straight trousers rather than the breeches or tights that harked back to the fifteenth century. It is interesting to contemplate where these loose pajama-like outfits came from in an age when the fashionable body was confined and displayed in tight doublets intricately tied to hose and leg-revealing breeches. Now, some four hundred years later, we can still recognize the commedia characters by their costumes, which have changed surprisingly little. Remarkably, too the costumes look acceptable to our twenty-first-century eyes—much more so than any breeches and tights would. Antoine Watteau, that wondrous recorder of theatrical performers at the beginning of the eighteenth century, portrayed Pierrot in paintings many times, but another of his works, *Iris*, a painting of children dating from sometime before 1720, may show the influence of the theatrical costume. It depicts a little boy, seated, playing a recorder-like pipe and wearing an altogether extraordinary outfit for its time, a silk jacket cut short, tailless, and loose, like the later men's frock (*le frac*), and straight-legged trousers that just cover his knee.

It was not until the 1770s that trousers moved up in society, and even then, they were for little boys only. But these little boys had powerful mothers, aristocratic and highly placed in that eighteenth-century world. European royal family portraits began to show little boys in straight trousers rather than knee breeches as early as 1778, as in *Four Grandchildren of Empress Maria Theresa* by Johann Zoffany. Five-year-old Prince Louis of Parma wears a silk hussar's suit, complete with decorative frogging closures on the little jacket, but with trousers that come to just above the ankles. As Diana De Marly suggests, wearing these at his age would imprint him for adulthood; he would want to wear them for the rest of his life, "and so would the rest of his generation."[3] The little hussar was first cousin to the dauphin of France, the son and heir of Marie Antoinette and Louis XVI. Several portraits of that doomed little boy dating from the 1780s, just before the Revolution, depict him wearing elegant versions of another little trouser outfit called a skeleton suit (or *matelot* in French). This had long straight trousers that buttoned onto a short, rather loose-fitting top, and was belted with a wide sash. It was worn with a crisp shirt underneath, with a ruffled open collar. Up until that time, until they were "breeched," little boys had worn the same skirts as their sisters, even if their outfits had more sober, masculine details. Thus, although white "baby dresses," which were also revolutionary, had appeared at mid-century, this was the first time children's clothing had broken away from the custom of dressing little boys to look like miniatures of their fathers. Although the royal children's outfits were made of silk and velvet, the basic form was wonderfully practical, and was adopted by many women for their little sons to wear in the years between diapers and breeches. The costume historian Doris Langley Moore called it "the greatest sartorial event of the eighteenth century" because "it was the first time comfort and convenience had been the basis of any fashion, at least in the present cycle of history."[4]

Scholars credit a number of influences for the emergence of this new clothing. Dating from the 1760s, Rousseau's philosophy of the natural man, with its attendant "back to nature" movement, called for, among other things, freeing children's bodies from tightly binding clothing. Other thinkers such as Winkelmann and Goethe rediscovered classical life and simplicity, and they too helped bring about this simpler form of children's clothing through the zeal of their followers.[5] In addition, John Locke had advocated "comfortable and functional clothing for children"; his influence may explain why it is generally accepted that the new skeleton suit was English in origin.[6] Locke notwithstanding, the style fit perfectly into the Anglomania that gripped all of Europe in the latter half of the eighteenth century. This fad for things English introduced many casual, sporting, country styles throughout the fashionable world of the time: men's frocks, redingotes, spencers, and so on, to say nothing of English styles of women's dress. Certainly by 1782, when Gainsborough painted a series of individual portraits of George III's family, including each of his thirteen children, three-year-old Prince Octavius was depicted wearing a skeleton suit.[7] Marie Antoinette, too, in all likelihood encouraged its use through her penchant for playacting at rural pleasures in her Petit Trianon at Versailles. Certainly, she was one of the first mothers to dress her son in it, and the numbers of family and mother-children portraits dating from when the dauphin was small would have ensured ready copying.

Ironically, the French Revolution's aversion to all things aristocratic also helped. In fact, the revolutionaries became known as the *sans-culottes*, meaning "without *culottes*," the French word for breeches, which were the trousers of the upper classes. Rejecting the knee breeches of fashion, the *sans-culottes* wore the straight-legged pants, or pantaloons, of the lower classes. Slowly, after the Revolution played itself out, pantaloons took over for men, taking more than a generation to finally nudge the knee breeches of the eighteenth century off the fashion map altogether. This history of bifurcation for men never ceased, then, but the garment took on a longer, looser, straight-legged form, often anchored under the shoe with a stirrup in the early years of the nineteenth century. It never looked back, after the 1820s becoming the menswear trouser of the past two centuries.

Little girls fell under influences of the "natural" movements of the late eighteenth century, too, although they did not have as far to go as boys did. The simple white baby dress had appeared among the upper classes, some-time around the 1750s, worn by toddlers of both sexes. It was new in its simplicity, and it was new in its fabric. Made out of cotton, it was easily washable, but was an expensive luxury in those years before the Industrial Revolution.[8] Many portraits of family groups show little children wearing this dress, some running and playing, distinguished by sex only by the color of the sash at the waist.[9] In the French style, girls wore pink sashes, boys blue. The little dresses invariably had a simple, unadorned neckline, straight short sleeves, and a long gathered skirt that fell almost to the ankle; three or four rows of growth tucks as a border provided the only other dec-oration on the dress. Later in the century it was this dress that little girls wore as companion outfits to the skeleton suits of their brothers. As the cen-tury advanced, the little sleeves became puffed, the waistline rose, and in general the dress foreshadowed the dress of adult women at the turn of the century. As the skirts became shorter and the muslin sheerer, active little girls (or perhaps their mothers) found that they needed something to pre-serve their modesty. It should be pointed out that up until this time, women had worn nothing under their chemises. Their underwear consisted of a simple chemise or shift, a pair of stays, and stockings rolled and tied at the knee with a ribbon. They believed that letting air circulate freely around the lower body was healthy. Drawers did exist, but really only for actresses on the stage, which of course gave the undergarments as dubious a reputation as their wearers had.[10] Even as early as the turn of the nineteenth century, long before Victorian prudery set in, exposing the legs was unthinkable. As Phillis and C. Willett Cunnington state, "For us there is a certain irony in the fact that the wearing of drawers by women [previously only a male garment] was considered extremely immodest."[11]

Sometime around 1803, particularly in England, trousers for girls, adapted from their brothers', appeared in the form of pantaloons that were meant to be worn underneath the lightweight dresses. At first they were hidden under the skirts, but as these rose, the pantaloons stayed ankle-length and finally became visible. These, then, were the first trousers actually meant to be seen that were worn by females in the West. Whereas the little boys' pantaloons were very plain and masculine, the little girls' had lace and tucks to tie them into the overall design of the dresses they accompanied. And as women's fashions followed the lightweight, high-waisted, airy styles of children's dress, women too began to wear pantaloons.[12] Finally, fashionable women were wearing trousers, if only for underwear. And not only were they English in origin, but they were introduced and worn for exercise as well, at least according to Pierre Dufay in 1906: "In 1807 there came from London the fashion for pantaloons for girls. Jumping exercises were practised in England in the girls' schools: it was for that that they wore the pantaloons."[13]

The Cunningtons tell a wonderful story about how these pantaloons gained their stamp of approval in society—and in the process give us a perfect example of fashion diffusion. (The story also reveals that royal teenagers two hundred years ago had much the same impulses teenagers have today.) Quoting a journal of 1811, they say "the invidious garment" was "being adopted by 'the dashers of the haut ton,' and when Royalty, in the person of Princess Charlotte, not merely wore them but freely revealed the fact, its future career was assured." The fifteen-year-old daughter of the Prince Regent, later George IV, she was very popular and "modern,"

> being forward, buckish about horses and full of exclamations very like
>
> swearing. She was sitting with her legs stretched out after dinner and
>
> shewed her drawers, which it seems she and most young women now

wear. Lady de Clifford said, "My dear Princess Charlotte, you shew your drawers." "I never do but where I can put myself at ease." "Yes, my dear, when you get in or out of a carriage." "I don't care if I do." "Your drawers are much too long." "I do not think so; the Duchess of Bedford's are much longer, and they are bordered with Brussels lace." "Oh," said Lady de Clifford in conclusion, "If she is to wear them, she does right to make them handsome."[14]

Some twenty years later, drawers were customary underwear for women, even though the fashion of the time had become much more elaborate and restrictive, for children as well as adults. Fabrics were heavier and stiffer than they had been at the turn of the century, and often they were dark and somber in color. By the 1840s, the upholstered look in clothing mirrored the burgeoning Victorian materialism that in turn reflected the rise of the prosperous industrial middle class by now enjoying the comfortable fruits of the Industrial Revolution. But the pantaloon, that sensible garment introduced in the lighter and more carefree period of the Empire and Regency to cover the extremities of little girls and women who insisted on wearing the sheer muslin dresses so popular at the time, remained. By now, it was a necessary part of women's underdress. Small wonder, then, that with its history of children's wear and underwear, it was rejected in the next decade, when, newly fabricated, it became the element of the bloomer costume that most offended.

The introduction of the pantaloon for children at the turn of the century was one influence that helped contemporary eyes accept the look. Another was the craze for "the Oriental," a term that included everything from the Middle East to Persia, India, and China. Although it came into full force in the eighteenth century, the contacts and therefore the links between Europe and the East had begun with the rise of Islam and the entry into Spain by the Moors in the eighth century. The Crusades brought back ideas, luxuries, and dress influences for the two hundred years of their duration, but the major link to the West came with the expansion of the Ottoman Turks to the borders of Europe, particularly Venice and Vienna, between 1380 and 1580.[15] At the beginning of the seventeenth century, two great European maritime nations, England and Holland, established their

East India companies, furthering the contacts and links with countries deeper within Asia. Although the English company grew and expanded throughout the century, it achieved stronger status only in the eighteenth century, when its power and authority in India deepened.[16] With the growing interest of the West in the East, primarily through its trade goods, things Eastern or Oriental became more and more fashionable. And the class that ran the company was the class that first adopted the look of the East—thus the eighteenth-century crazes for Chinese porcelain, for chocolate, coffee, and tea, for cotton chintzes and palempores,[17] even for operas set in exotic locales, such as Mozart's *Abduction from the Seraglio* (1782). It meant, also, a fascination with the clothes of the Orient.

Many upper-class Europeans had their portraits painted wearing clothing influenced or borrowed from countries east of Europe. Turkish dress elements such as the turban and the wrap coat and pantaloons worn with a wide sash encased English and French bodies, as captured by the leading portraitists of the day, among them Liotard, Aved, Gainsborough, Reynolds, and Copley.[18] Other artists, such as Angelica Kauffmann, painted more general subjects while dressing their sitters in *turquerie*.[19] It had vaulted into English society's awareness when Lady Mary Wortley Montagu wrote of her travels in Turkey in the early eighteenth century. She not only described the clothing of Turkish women but also brought some of it home and had her portrait painted wearing it, including the trousers that were so much a part of Turkish women's dress. According to Aileen Ribeiro, she set the fashion not just for portraits *à la turque* but for masquerade *à la turque* as well.[20] The foreign dress lent itself to fashion. Elements of it, mixed with European styles, appeared in fashion plates of the late eighteenth century under the guise of "circassiennes" or "levites," and turbans became part of women's fashion wear towards the end of the century. As for men, they relished their undress, their *déshabillé*, in the form of caps or turbans to cover their shaved heads at home when their wigs were put aside, and their "nightgowns" or banyans, which they wore for leisure for at least a century and a half.[21] Samuel Pepys, for example, noted in his diary entry of March 30, 1666, that he wore his India gown for his sitting with the painter John Hales.[22] All this, of course, argues for the enormous popularity of a new and different look.

By the nineteenth century, after Napoleon's incursions into Africa, the French painters Ingres and Delacroix captured the exoticism and mystery of North Africa and its culture and customs, including enticing portrayals of the seraglio or harem. Ingres began as early as 1808 with his painting *The Valpinçon Bather*, which, though of a nude, strongly suggests the Middle East through the turban wrapped around the sitter's hair. (This pose and even the striped cloth was revisited fifty-four years later, when Ingres was eighty-two, in his famous painting *The Turkish Bath*.) Another well-known work was his *Odalisque with a Slave* of 1840. Whereas the main subject was, once again, nude, the servants wore the clothing of North Africa, complete with Turkish trousers. While Ingres painted nudes, Delacroix, his contemporary and one of the earliest artists to espouse the Romantic, depicted the clothed body. He visited Spain, Morocco, and Turkey in 1832, and returned to France with a portfolio of watercolors and drawings that he later used as the basis for some one hundred paintings. He documented in Romantic, vigorous, and imaginative works the dress of both virile men and languorous women, rich in color and exotic in detail. One, *Algerian Women in Their Apartments* (1834), clearly shows the Turkish trouser, with its baggy, full pants gathered at the ankle or the knee and worn beneath a tunic or bolero. It was that trouser, of course, that provided the model for the more generically applied term, used in a broader sense throughout the rest of the century, to describe any gathered trouser form. And these paintings, shown in Paris, would have been seen widely by the people who mattered most for our purposes—the people who could influence fashion.

Orientalism in its newer interpretation had crossed the English Channel during the early nineteenth century, taking its most remarkable form in the whimsical and exotic architectural excess of the Regency period, the Prince Regent's Royal Pavilion at Brighton (1808). The Orientalism adopted at this time, far from being a true borrowing of another culture's design, was instead a lavish and jubilant amalgam of all influences from points east (or south) of Europe. As we have seen, this movement had started in the later years of the eighteenth century, but it took flight in the fancy dress balls that were a popular form of aristocratic entertainment during this time and throughout the early years of Queen Victoria's reign, while Prince Albert was still alive. Ladies were recorded as having worn Turkish costume, daring in the extreme because of the trousers they were required to wear for "authenticity."

Here, then, we see that trousers for women in the guise of Mrs. Bloomer's reform dress did not just appear out of nowhere at mid-century, only to be dismissed by a narrow-minded and judgmental public because they were too new, too shocking. The idea had been around for a long time. It was the application of that idea to women's daily dress, as we have seen, that caused all the problems.

THE RISE OF INTEREST IN
Exercise for Women

As the fascination for the Oriental underwent a change with the onset of Romanticism, the simplicity in women's dress that had characterized the more carefree and lusty Empire and Regency periods eroded, to be finally lost in the 1820s. With its passing, the concept of freedom of movement in women's clothing disappeared too. Instead, serious corsetry took the place of the emphatic cantilevering of the bosom that had sufficed in the years of the high waist, while new layers of underskirts began to shape the fuller skirts that were to continue to expand in size over the next half century. The new styles of clothing, more physically restraining, more stylized, and decidedly heavier, gave the new ideal woman her quintessential look of constrained and covered modesty. Unlike her mother and grandmother, she was demure and spiritual, a model of gentleness and passivity, virtue and motherhood. She was elevated to her pedestal as the cult of true womanhood flowered. As Geoffrey Squire put it, by 1837, the year Victoria ascended the throne, "men were not to be subdued, but became deferential. . . . The bounce was quite gone, replaced by a sensitive fragility."[1]

Throughout the mid-century years, popular literature reinforced the philosophy supporting the cult. Charles Dickens's early novels invariably described the heroines as gentle, passive, lovely, aristocratic in bearing if not birth, and often tragic. Little Dorrit and *David Copperfield*'s Dora are classic examples of the sweet, somewhat dull, and decidedly asexual ideal.

Dickens and other authors attached moralistic connotations to the livelier, deeper, and more complex women in the novels of the period: the women of exposed sexuality, such as Lady Dedwood of *Bleak House* and Becky Sharp in *Vanity Fair*, invariably came to a bad end. Stories and articles in the women's magazines that proliferated, notably, in America, the enduring *Godey's Lady's Book*—which debuted, under the leadership of Sarah Josepha Hale, with Queen Victoria in 1837—again and again reiterated the passivity, the nobility of spirit, and the gentility that characterized the cult of true womanhood. Under the watchful, guiding commentary of its editor, generations of women sought the true path of duty and motherhood, women's proper "sphere."[2]

As the image of the new ideal of womanhood solidified, mannerisms as well as clothing reflected the change. Women affected an appearance of delicacy, with pale complexion and slightness of figure, encouraged by the new, exquisitely engineered corsetry which now covered the entire midsection from the chest to the lower hips and sharply defined a waist that had been overlooked for decades. Dieting, too, became a fad among young women. A favorite method was to drink vinegar water and to pick at one's food (probably not too difficult to do if the vinegar water went first).[3] Tight-lacing led to ailments such as "palpitation, the vapors, and swooning,"[4] and rendered active movement all but impossible. The look of the 1840s had traveled a long way from the revealing, flirtatious, and overtly sexual clothing of the previous generation. Geoffrey Squire cannot be improved on for capturing "the dullest decade in the history of feminine dress":

> The last vestige of the expansive sleeve hung modestly about the wrist, the upper section above the elbow encircled only by a few delicate frills or close set gauging. The corset was cut much longer in the waist, and its curves were drawn out into shallow, sinuous lines which moulded the bust tightly like the calyx of a still-closed flower. By 1840, the bonnet, its brim much reduced, closed closely round the face in a narrow inverted U. The hair, centrally parted, was plastered down with "Bandoline," seemingly painted on to the perfect oval of the head, and from ear-level it dripped into long forlorn "spaniel" ringlets. Timidity and helpless resignation were emphasized by the

binding of the arms to the body in a shawl; exactly placed about the points of the shoulders, it muffled the figure and carried the eye down the billowing figure without a break. . . . [T]he gaze slides down the drooping shoulders, then slithers the length of the elongated torso, over the gently padded hips and on to the heavy dragging skirts, which were supported by a burden of innumerable petticoats. The plump, cheeky little girls of the preceding years had been transformed into enervated, shy, serious adolescents, slender and gazelle-like.

It was, according to Squire, an insipid, mediocre, "entirely middle-class epoch. . . . Hardly an atmosphere to encourage invention or emulation."[5] Oddly enough, though, perhaps even because the times were so uninspiring, invention and innovation abounded in the 1840s.

An early hint at revolution appeared in *Godey's* in July 1841. In an article titled "How To Begin," Sarah Hale wrote about educating daughters and the importance of "physical education . . . for the constitution," a "department of training children [that] is, in our country, more neglected than any other." She continues:

> We lately met with a little book, written by a physician of Glasgow, Scotland, which contained many sensible observations, as Scotch works usually do. It was entitled—RULES FOR INVIGORATING THE CONSTITUTION. . . .
>
> In the first place, females, from their earliest years, should be allowed those sports and amusements in the open air, so necessary to the proper development of their bodies, and which are now confined entirely to boys. Instead of being compelled to walk demurely with measured steps, like so many matrons, they should be encouraged in running and romping even, at suitable times; and that the motions of their limbs may be unconstrained, their dress should be always loose and easy.
>
> Until girls are fourteen or fifteen years old, they should be allowed to play in the open air at least *six hours* every day, when the season and weather will permit. They should be allowed to run, leap, throw the

ball, and play at battledore, as they please. All these exercises call the different muscles into action, strengthen the limbs, and impart a healthy tone to the different organs; the blood circulates freely, the nervous system is invigorated, and the redundant fluids are driven off by perspiration. The most suitable dress is unquestionably that which is called Turkish, consisting of pantalettes or trowsers, and a short frock (the latter to be brought up sufficiently high on the bosom to prevent the exposure of the shoulders) and the covering of the head should be light and cool—a straw hat answers the purpose very well.[6]

This, ten years before the bloomer.

The unnamed Scottish doctor was a proponent of a growing movement to introduce physical culture to the population at large. (Elizabeth Blackwell, as we saw in Part One, was another.) Although the 1830s and 1840s were perhaps the low point in the history of exercise for women, as early as 1826 a Boston teacher, William Bentley Fowle, had attempted (and failed) to find a precedent for girls to use before introducing a new system of German gymnastics that had been devised for boys only. In making this attempt, he commented with some insight, "It seemed as if the sex had been thought unworthy of an effort to improve their physical powers." Eleven years later, in 1837, the *Boston Medical and Surgical Journal* still had cause to chide parents for slighting their daughters' physical education.[7] Interestingly, though, an illustration in *Atkinson's Casket* from 1832 had shown a young woman practicing "female calisthenics," wearing a costume virtually the same as the one described by the Scottish doctor in 1841.[8] So even as the sages, medical authorities, and educators were advocating the cause of exercise over a period of a decade or more, it seems that some women had already taken the matter into their own hands. Generally, though, progress came slowly.

In attempting to adapt German exercises for girls, the Boston teacher probably patterned his series on that of Friedrich Ludwig Jahn, one of two early exercise leaders to gain an international following. Jahn's famous work *Die Deutsche Turnkunst*, published in 1816, was a German nomenclature for exercise, calling it *Turner* rather than using the more accepted "gymnastics," which had a Greek root. From this, the *Turnverein*, or gym-

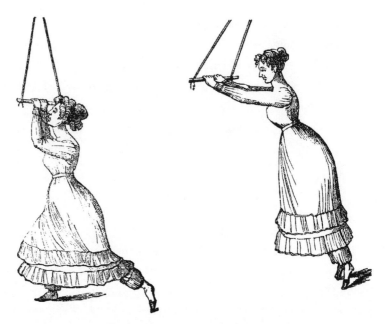

Female calisthenics. *Atkinson's Casket*, April 1832, 187. Courtesy of Boston Athenaeum.

nastic societies, grew; the participants and the system both became known as "turners." The other leader, the Swede, Per Ling, opened the Royal Gymnastics Central Institute of Stockholm in 1814, but it was his son, Hjalmar, who turned the emphasis of gymnastics towards education. Although physical education at first benefited only boys, other teachers gradually adapted the systems for girls, so that when the educator Catharine Beecher visited a Russian seminary at mid-century, she was able on her return to describe in glowing terms the "more than 900 girls from noble families [who] were being trained in Ling's calisthenics."[9] In the United States, German immigrants had brought their *Turner* with them, and practiced them in their own communities. But until Dio Lewis made gymnastics fashionable in America in the 1860s, few educators promoted this form of exercise, and certainly not for girls.

Catharine Beecher had been delighted to see calisthenics for girls performed en masse in Russia, even if it was some twenty years since she had first insisted on them as part of her curriculum in her schools in the United States. Such was her influence and importance in her time that she played a prominent role in introducing calisthenics as part of girls' education. In order to understand how she accomplished this, it helps to know more about her. Indeed, no account of the history of women's education in the United States can be meaningful without some reference to Catharine Beecher, the eldest of the remarkable Beecher family mentioned in Part One. As noted previously, the Beechers' careers centered on the church from the period of the Second Great Awakening very early in the century, from father Lyman through the sons and sons-in-law. The Beechers were very typically middle class, but gained acceptance at higher levels of society because of their importance in the religious life of the era as well-known orators, preachers, and ministers. Later, the women of the family achieved even greater fame in literary and educational circles.

In the early decades of the century, the church was one of the few avenues by which the middle class could achieve upward mobility, but only men of the family were allowed this entree. It was an ironic point, and one not lost on Catharine, that men were able to gain significant positions at lofty levels through the auspices of the church solely because the women of the republic had come forward by the hundreds of thousands to swell the growing religious movement in what has been called "the feminization of American religion."[10] The church was one of the only acceptable places for social participation outside the home for a middle-class woman. In addition, she might even find a measure of influence there. Her position as supporter of the church and of its clergy had its own merit. Religious activism for women depended, however, on the "implicit bargain between clergymen and women parishioners" that women would avoid seeking leadership roles. "As long as a woman kept her 'proper place,' a tract society pamphlet explained in 1823, she might exert 'almost any degree of influence she pleases.'"[11] In other words, the church was regarded as part of "women's sphere." The Second Great Awakening, then, was a mass movement of women led by a select few, all men, all clergy. And of these the Beecher men were among the most prominent.

Catharine Beecher, a determined and competitive spirit brought up by a leader in a family of leaders and seeking a leadership role herself, was aware that her destiny lay apart from the church simply because of the accident of gender. She elected, therefore, to achieve her success in the field of education. Her chosen path led her to found the Hartford Female Seminary in

1824, and to carry her influence to the West, to Cincinnati in 1832. She fervently believed in education for women, understanding perhaps more graphically than many, because of the family of achievers in which she grew up, that for women to attain any kind of equality, they must be educated equally to men. She was very much a product of her generation and family, however, and therefore her view of equality was one of "separate but equal." Indeed, not only was women's sphere a concept she accepted, but it became the rallying point of her crusade for women's education as well. She believed that women should be educated to educate others, and she encouraged the formation of many teacher-training institutions around the country. The subjects that women were to be educated in were all related to women's sphere. She wanted nothing less than a profession for women that would have equal importance not just to motherhood but to those of men: the ministry, medicine, and the law. She sold her plan by arguing, first, that women were more naturally attuned to children, and second, and perhaps even more telling, that they could work for half a man's salary or less.[12] It was an argument that few communities could resist.

To disseminate her ideas (and also to earn a living), she wrote the monumental guide that was to be used widely over the next forty years and more, *A Treatise on Domestic Economy*, first published in Boston in 1841 and reprinted almost every year until 1856. Subtitled "for the use of young ladies at home and at school," it was clearly a teaching tool for the young ladies she taught. But its wider success was overwhelming, and it established her as the outstanding authority on all things pertaining to the American home. Katherine Kish Sklar, Beecher's biographer, refers to the work as the nineteenth-century equivalent to Dr. Benjamin Spock's *Baby and Child Care* of a century later.[13] In it, Beecher created and defined a new profession for women, the domestic economist. Centered firmly in the home, she was in command of every conceivable aspect of domestic activity. Her orderly approach to home management paved the way for the later educators who transformed it into household science or home economics, a field that, during its century of existence, sought to educate young women in all aspects of family, home, and domestic management while giving them pride in their homemaker roles.[14] The *Treatise*, then, not only defined the role young women would play in the home, bringing to it an aura of professionalism, but also offered practical advice on how to accomplish the multifaceted aspects of the job. American women, Beecher believed, were united by their dedication to the role.[15] In short, Beecher clearly defined women's sphere and gave it respectabilty.

Like others of her time, Beecher believed that the fundamental reason for educating girls was to create a nation of strong wives and mothers to raise and educate the next generations of American citizens. "Let the women of the country be made virtuous and intelligent, and the men will certainly be the same," she wrote. "The proper education of a man decides the welfare of an individual; but educate a woman and the interests of a whole family are secured." In spite of her staunch support of the potential power of women in society, however, she was forced to admit that a great difficulty "peculiar to American women, is a delicacy of constitution, which renders them early victims to disease and decay." She blamed this "debility of constitution . . . on the mismanagement of early life."[16] To counteract this poor beginning of a girl's life, she advocated adequate exercise, proper diet and clothing, cleanliness, and fresh air—all, interestingly enough, innovations in her time but still entirely recognizable as necessary in ours. She railed against corsets, asserting that they distorted the body and prevented exercise, and she created her own sets of exercises, even providing illustrations showing how to do them. She published these and her other ideas on promoting good health in *Letters to the People on Health and Happiness* (1854) and *Physiology and Calisthenics for Schools and Families* (1856). Beecher understood the importance of such early training and healthful endeavor because she herself was a victim of "female invalidism" throughout her adult life. She believed firmly in the virtues of the water cure, a popular form of treatment from the 1840s to the 1880s. As Sklar tells us, during this period "213 water-cure centers emerged to treat a predominantly female clientele, and Catharine Beecher was among their most enthusiastic patrons."[17] It is here, with her books on health and exercise, with her advocacy of the spas, which combined treatment and exercise, and with her calisthenics program "for schools and families," that Beecher becomes of special interest to us. It is particularly significant that she introduced calisthenics for girls as early as the 1830s in her Western Seminary in Cincinnati.[18]

The links between Catharine Beecher's calisthenics and a specific exercise dress (such as the bloomer) are tenuous. Her own illustrations from

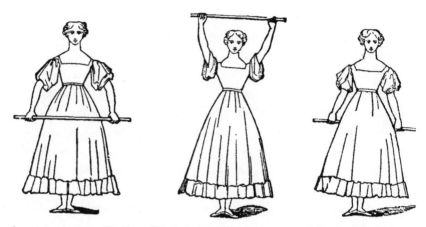

Correct exercise dress. *The Young Girl's Book of Healthful Amusements and Exercises* (New York: Kiggins and Kellogg, n.d., but probably late 1820s). Thanks to Susan Greene of American Costume Studies.

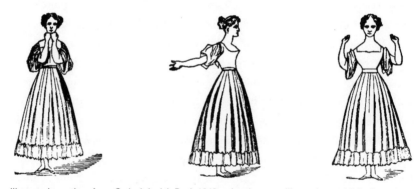

Illustrated exercises from *Godey's Lady's Book*, 1848, using the same illustrations published some ten to twenty years earlier in *The Young Girl's Book*.

1856 show a sort of amalgam of a dress more like one published in *Godey's* in 1848, which in turn borrowed directly from an even earlier book dating from the late 1820s or 1830.[19] It had a higher-than-natural waist, a bell skirt shortened to above the ankle, and short sleeves that are full and fall as the arms are raised, all characteristic of fashionable dress from the very late 1820s and early 1830s. Significantly, it differs from the earlier model in that the young woman in Beecher's illustration wears pantalettes underneath, more in keeping with the exercise dresses we have already seen, or even the bloomer. But the ties to the bloomer may consist of more than the little pantalettes lurking beneath the skirt. It seems that Elizabeth Smith Miller (daughter of the temperance and abolitionist reformer Gerrit Smith) visited her cousin Elizabeth Cady Stanton on her return from her honeymoon in Europe, wearing the prototype outfit that she had had made for her travels after seeing similar clothing worn at health spas and retreats for women in Europe. As we saw in Part One, Amelia Bloomer herself stated that both Stanton and Miller wore the costume before she herself did, so this much of the story is true. Documentation is scant, but a number of accounts relate this link between Elizabeth Smith Miller and the European spas. It is clear that these health retreats existed both in Europe and in America, and it is to the ones at home that Catharine Beecher escaped when necessary. Elizabeth Cady Stanton, towards the end of her life, reminisced that the bloomer costume was worn by "many patients in sanatariums, whose names I cannot recall," and also by "farmer's [sic] wives, skaters, gymnasts, tourists."[20] And recall the Scottish doctor cited in Godey's who advocated Turkish trousers for young girls for exercise. Although Catharine Beecher does not specifically mention clothing, other than to demand a loosening of corsets, it is interesting to speculate that the same Turkish trousers might have been worn in those female-populated spas in the United States. If we are to believe Elizabeth Cady Stanton, they certainly were. What is clear is that Beecher's sponsoring of physical exercise must have led to an awareness of a need for suitable clothing. And to judge by her illustrations, the drawers that had become necessary for girls' underwear answered that need.

Catharine Beecher was only one of many who believed that women's future role depended greatly on their further education. The early years of the nineteenth century saw the establishment of several schools for young women—mostly "academies" and "seminaries." Emma Willard's Troy Seminary for Women, the first endowed school for women, founded in 1821, was an early example. It catered to the "ambitious middle classes" and became a model for teacher-training schools of the future. Although progressive in demanding higher standards and original thought, it still remained well within the expectations of women's sphere. According to Emma Willard's sister, Almira Hart Lincoln Phelps, who was also an educator, its main purpose was to turn the students into "better daughters, wives, and sisters; better qualified for usefulness in every path within the sphere of female exertions."[21] Its influence was long-term; unlike Catharine Beecher's schools, which lasted only a few years, it still exists today as a highly regarded prep school.

Two other women also sought new kinds of schools for young women. Zilpah Grant and Mary Lyon met in 1821, the year the Troy Seminary was founded, at Joseph Emerson's school in Byfield, Massachusetts, where they were both students. Grant, three years older, mentored Mary Lyon, who adored her and learned from her. Out of their relationship developed a lasting and devoted friendship that would lead first to Grant's Ipswich Academy and ultimately to Lyon's Mount Holyoke Seminary, which would influence women's higher education in this country for the rest of the century and beyond.[22] Mary Lyon borrowed ideas from both the Troy Seminary and Ipswich Academy, but went further than either. She wanted more rigorous academic standards that would give women an education equal to those at the colleges for young men. She also wanted—needed—an endowed institution, but after failing to find support in Ipswich, she moved west to a village in the Connecticut River valley, South Hadley, near Amherst, where Joseph Emerson had settled when he took a position at Amherst College. Her goal was to prepare girls for wider social roles (often as teachers or wives of missionaries), but because she was a product of her era, both the methods and the expectations were within the framework of women's sphere. Echoing Beecher, she declared, "Our future statesmen and rulers, ministers and missionaries must come inevitably under the moulding hand of the female."[23] Here she found the support she needed, and was able to open Mount Holyoke Seminary in 1837 with a curriculum and student life reflective of its time, a curious amalgam of high academic standards, domestic preparation, and strong piety. She thus provided a prototype for women's higher education that was emulated over and over throughout the country as schools for women opened. And exercise was important from the beginning.

"Exercise," Lyon wrote in 1837, "is worth very much more than I anticipated, especially in the winter. The daily work brings one hour of regular exercise coming every day. . . . The exercise is particularly fitted to the constitution of females."[24] The "daily work" that was particularly fitting, it must be said, was domestic work, incorporated into the students' routine as policy to save the expense of hiring servants in order to cut costs of the girls' education. As Lyon relates, each student spent at least one hour every day on some chore in the college, whether sweeping, scrubbing, setting and clearing tables, washing dishes, baking, doing the laundry—everything, in fact, but cooking.[25] But just in case this activity was not quite enough, the seminary's Book of Duties reminded that "The young ladies are to be required to walk one mile per day until the snow renders it desirable to specify time instead of distance, when three-quarters of an hour is the time required."[26]

An early student in the school, Lucy T. Goodale, wrote lively and engaging letters home to her family, vividly describing her life there. In 1838 she reported: "The young ladies here are divided into three classes in calisthenics, one for each spaceway. They exercise every evening from half past eight to nine o'clock. This gives them new vigor for study the remaining hour before retiring. In addition to this and running up and down stairs, Miss Lyon wished to have us take a walk every morning before breakfast. So you see she wishes not to have us suffer for want of air and exercise."[27] Or from want of things to fill their time. The rising bell rang at 5 AM, and chores as well as the invigorating walk were completed before breakfast, which was at 7:00.

The calisthenics Lucy mentioned were a part of the curriculum from the first year the school opened. Mary Lyon herself wrote out the instructions and gathered them in a small publication, *Calisthenic Exercises.*[28] Contemporaries regarded Mount Holyoke as most unusual, even peculiar, in demanding any kind of exercise other than dignified walking. So it is of little surprise in this pious Congregational New England atmosphere, where dancing was anathema, that a strong note of defensiveness colored the admonition in the "Teachers' Book of Duties": "Care should be taken that the exercise does not become like dancing in the impression it makes on observers."[29] To counteract any misconception, the school replaced the original Lyon exercises with Dio Lewis's program in 1862. The earlier calisthenics certainly could not have been too strenuous; no doubt they were "fitting to the constitution of females." The school did not even require any special dress for them, nor did it make any suggestion about the removal of stays. But the more regimented curriculum of calisthenics put forth by Lewis brought about a new interest, even a vogue for exercise for both men and women in the 1860s, which lasted well beyond that decade.

The entire question of exercise programs in the United States had been a somewhat hit or miss affair, based on Jahn's German *Turner* format, the Lings' Swedish exercises, or the sets of calisthenics for women such as those devised by Mary Lyon and espoused by Catharine Beecher. All that changed with Dio Lewis and his *New Gymnastics for Men, Women, and Children*, published in 1862.

Dio (short for Diocletian) Lewis became what we would call today the guru of exercise in the 1860s. Indeed, had he lived 150 years later, his personality, drive, and methods might very well have qualified him for the highly paid, highly visible career of a motivational speaker, sideshow snake oil overtones and all, as one story about him suggests. When an early Oberlin College physical education professor, Delphine Hanna, asked him in the 1880s whether there might be a scientific basis for the need for exercise, she was shocked when he shot back: "You don't need a scientific basis. People want to be hum-bugged."[30] But even as he might have been "humbugging" all along, he, like his descendants today, struck a chord and developed a huge and devoted following.

As he became aware that the various exercise systems developed earlier in the century appealed only to the young, the fit, the muscular, and the male, Lewis began to consider other possibilities as the movement gained momentum at mid-century. He spent eight years on the lecture circuit in the 1850s, later recalling:

> During the eight years of lecturing the spare hours were devoted to the invention of a new system of gymnastics. The old, or German gymnastics, the one so common throughout our country, was obviously not adapted to the classes most needing artificial training. Athletic young men, who alone succeeded in the feats of the gymnasium, were already provided for. Boat clubs, ball clubs and other sports furnished them in considerable part with the means of muscular training. But old men, fat men, feeble men, young boys and females of all ages—the class most needing physical training—were not drawn to the old-fashioned gymnasium. The few attempts that had been made to introduce these classes to that institution had uniformly and signally failed. The system itself was wrong.[31]

Reading this today, women might bristle at being clumped into the same category as males who were old, fat, feeble, or adolescent. But that would be to lose sight of the fact that Lewis devised a system that would have an even greater impact in this country than the earlier German or Swedish systems, and he automatically included women in the design from the start. However overpowering his showmanship qualities, he was an advocate for women and exercise throughout his career.

After his eight years "on the road," he introduced his new exercises in Boston in 1860, and in the following year founded there the Normal Institute for Physical Education (the Essex Street Gymnasium), a training school for teachers of "the New System." It was certainly not the first of its kind ever, as he liked to claim, but it nevertheless was the first of its kind in the United States. With the opening of his school, he became Dr. Lewis, M.D., Professor of Gymnastics. Not surprisingly, the M.D. was honorary (it is not entirely clear from where), but used ever after. The professorship was valid at least in his own school. According to an 1861 article, "Gymnastics," in the *Atlantic Monthly*:

> It would be unpardonable . . . not to speak a good word for the favorite hobby of the day—Dr. Lewis and his system of gymnastics, or, more properly, of calisthenics. Dr. Winship [a contemporary who advocated exercise for building strength by weight lifting] had done all that was needed in some apostleship of severe exercises, and there was wanting some man with a milder hobby, perfectly safe for a lady to drive. . . . [I]t is just what is wanted for multitudes of persons who find or fancy the real gymnasium unsuited to them. It will especially render service to female pupils, so far as they practise it; for the accustomed gymnastic exercises seem never yet to have been rendered attractive to them, on any large scale, and with any permanency.[32]

Here we learn a number of things. First, gymnasiums were being built to encourage men's exercise during this time, but it was thought that women might not feel comfortable coming to them. This may be interpreted from several points of view. The most obvious (to a woman, anyway) would be that, in all likelihood, men had no interest in admitting women to their gyms, which at this time were few and far between. Later, when gyms were more numerous, schedules were worked out for separate hours for men and women. But in the early 1860s, at the start of the Civil War, such was not yet the case. After the war, when reformers tried to rebuild from the horrors of the previous four years, they stressed the need for exercise to keep men strong, even more so than before the war. It was then that the YMCA branched out into a wider focus. Established in 1844 as an evangelical movement to aid young men in England who were at risk because of the dire conditions brought about by the Industrial Revolution, the Young Men's Christian Association expanded to North America in 1851. Its facilities included gyms and eventually, by the 1880s, swimming pools. The YMCA represents in microcosm the growth of "muscular Christianity," the movement linking exercise and evangelical religion that seems to have played such a large role in nineteenth-century society. It figured prominently even at Mount Holyoke Seminary, as Mary Lyon's admonitions prove. A second interpretation the 1861 article suggests is that women were better off doing their exercise in the privacy of their own homes. Exercise was new to them, it was unattractive, and it was hard to keep at. Why bother going to a gym to do it? When we compare this author's subtly patronizing tone with Dio Lewis's exuberant support of women, we begin to realize just how unusual Lewis was for his time.

Soon after Lewis opened his Normal School, he conducted a school for girls, from 1864 to 1867, in Lexington, Massachusetts; Catharine Beecher was, for a while, one of the lecturers. It burned down after three years, but throughout its short existence some three hundred students enrolled there. The school, like its founder, was unusual, offering a decidedly original curriculum (but, even so, with an echo of Mary Lyon) and attracting students who were perhaps outside the norm. In Lewis's own words:

> [The school] drew together a company of bright girls, with delicate constitutions, such girls as could not bear the exclusively mental pressure of the ordinary school. . . . The girls went to bed at half-past eight every evening. They rose early in the morning and went out to walk, which walk was repeated during the day. They ate only twice a day, and of very plain, nourishing food. They took off their corsets. They

exercised twice a day, half an hour, in gymnastics, and danced an hour about three times a week. This was the general course, and upon this regimen they rapidly improved. The gymnastics exercises proved invaluable, but the nine hours in bed, I believe, played a still more important part.[33]

Girls were measured on entrance and were found to increase in girth and decrease in weight.

Lewis's *New Gymnastics* was reprinted and largely revised in 1868. In it he not only laid out the exercises, he commented on the order of doing them, the value of doing them, and the clothing to be worn while doing them. The illustrations, line drawings or "cuts," depicted both men and women. In describing the costume for exercise, Lewis defined the difference between adapted fashionable dress and real exercise clothing:

Men and boys exercising in an occasional class simply remove the coat and exercise in ordinary dress; but a costume made of flannel, in the style seen in the cuts, is better for regular work.

In the ladies' costume, perfect liberty about the waist and shoulders is *the* desideratum. Many ladies imagine if the skirt be short it constitutes the gymnastic costume. The skirt should be short, but this is of little importance compared with the fit of the dress about the upper half of the body. The belt should be several inches larger than the waist, and the dress about the shoulders very loose. The best waist is a regular Garibaldi, with the seam on the shoulder so short that the armhole seam is drawn up to the top of the shoulder-joint. The stockings should, for cold weather, be thick woollen, and for appearance sake another pair of cotton stockings be worn over them; the shoes strong, with broad soles and low heels.[34]

It is interesting to compare his description of the approved outfit with the illustrations in the book. The skirt was indeed short for the day. But Lewis never mentions the bloomer worn underneath it, clearly visible in most of the cuts. Perhaps these are the "cotton stockings" worn over the

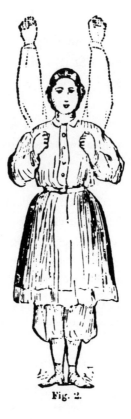

Dio Lewis's gymnastic dress, 1862, echoes both the bloomer costume and the bathing dress of the 1850s and 1860s. Dio Lewis, *The New Gymnastics for Men, Women, and Children*, 10th ed. (Boston: Fields, Osgood & Co., 1869).

Fig. 2.

"thick woollen" ones. And "for appearance sake" is no doubt the period's modest way of insisting that a woman's "limbs" remain thoroughly covered, and discreetly unmentioned. The Garibaldi, a fashion staple of the 1860s, as noted earlier, was the perfect answer to the need for a loose, roomy top that would allow the arms to move freely without yanking it out of the skirt waistband.[35]

A photograph from Mount Holyoke College depicting a calisthenics team in 1865 shows Dio Lewis's influence. Here we see students dressed in exactly the costume he illustrated and described. The skirts are short, falling just below the knee, revealing bloomers below the hem of the skirts; stockings fill the gap between the bloomers and the boot tops. The sleeves are full and gathered from dropped shoulder seams (typical of the 1860s, but unlike Lewis's suggested higher seam) and are attached to baggy bodices that allow the wearer the necessary room to swing her arms. Waists

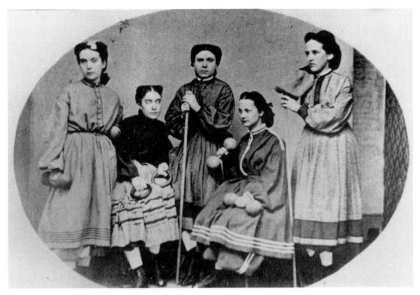

Gymnastic team, Mount Holyoke College, 1865. All five wear personalized and probably homemade versions of Dio Lewis's gymnastic dress. Courtesy of Mount Holyoke College Special Collections and Archive.

are loose, gathered, bloused. There is not a hint of the body-hugging clothing that was fashionable at that period, or that would have indicated the presence of corsets underneath. But in no way are the outfits uniform. Each gymnastic dress represented a personal choice of color, individual style within the general guidelines, and trim. Even the fabric seems to have been a personal choice. We learn why this was so, and where at least some of the dresses came from, in a letter Margaret Etta Noble wrote to her parents: "I cut out a waist of a gymnastic dress for one of the girls today and it fitted real nice."[36] So popular did the dresses become that they were soon a staple in the fashion magazines that offered patterns, often being described as suitable for either bathing or gymnastics. For example, the varieties of styles and trim can be seen in illustrations from *La Mode Illustrée* of 1871.[37] These are for children between the ages of six and twelve, but they fit the description in *The New Gymnastics* perfectly.

Of course, if exercise was now fashionable, one could be sure that *Godey's* would note the trend—especially since it had been an advocate of exercise for decades. But according to *Godey's*, Dio Lewis's dress had taken on some decidedly non-utilitarian features. One wonders, in fact, just what purposes the dresses would have been put to, or who would be joining the wearer in order to appreciate the luxuriousness of her outfit. In January 1864 *Godey's* described "some very attractive costumes for the always healthful, now popular light parlour gymnastics." The article continues:

> One very tasteful dress was of Russian gray Empress cloth, a fine quality trimmed with leaf-green velvet; the depth of velvet at the bottom of the skirt was about eight inches, cut in at the upper edge in two patterns, alternating, which gave style and variety to the skirt, and also to the body and sleeves whenever applied. The edge of the velvet is finished in the tiniest gold braid; then a jet, and then another gold braid, the two last put on in pattern. The body was a plaited [pleated] Garibaldi, with deep yoke pointed in front, and extending to the waist, and finished with cut velvet, and braided to agree with the skirt. The sleeve was in the prevailing mode, without seams inside of the arm, but ingeniously confined to the wrist, and adapted to the costume. Wide Turkish pants of the same completes the dress.
>
> Another pretty costume for a young lady was a "Tartan" plaid skirt, with scarlet trimmings, the upper edge cut in pattern, and braided with narrow black velvet. Waist of black Empress cloth, with scarlet yoke, and a rolling collar; an embroidered linen collar, "Cavalier" style, and black silk tie finished the neck. Full pants in black Empress cloth is worn with this suit.[38]

Clearly, *Godey's* was more interested in the fashionable details of the outfits than in their suitability even for "light parlour gymnastics."

Thus, in spite of Dio Lewis's guidelines for exercise clothing, a uniform dress for gymnastic wear was still very much a thing of the future. But with his suggestions, and given the popularity of the activity, which for women could be done in seclusion at home, the prototype had been introduced, and women who wished to participate enthusiastically embraced it.

INNOVATION AT
Wellesley

A Uniform for Crew

THE YEARS BETWEEN DIO LEWIS'S *NEW GYMNASTICS* AND SENDA BEREN-son's introduction of basketball for women in the early 1890s saw a con-tinuation of the interest in sporting activities and exercise. They also witnessed a slowly growing acceptance of the notion of women's higher education. Schools for women, some of them connected to existing men's colleges (Barnard and Columbia, Radcliffe and Harvard, Sophie Newcomb and Tulane) and founded during the last thirty or so years of the nine-teenth century, offered girls an education supposedly comparable to their brothers'. Most of the schools appeared in the 1880s and later, and all of them profited from the pioneers: Mount Holyoke (1837), Vassar (1865), and Wellesley and Smith (both 1875). All of these early schools for women encouraged physical exercise from the start, but only Vassar stipulated a specific uniform—and that disappeared soon after. But between the new exercise dress worn at Mount Holyoke in the 1860s, based on Dio Lewis's model, and the skirtless basketball outfit adopted at Smith in the 1890s, another sort of non-fashionable informal dress appeared. Evidence of it still exists in photographs from Wellesley and Mount Holyoke, the earliest dating from 1879. It consisted of a bloused shirt reminiscent of Dio Lewis's exercise dress, worn with a long skirt. I can find no evidence of it in *The Delineator*, that invaluable magazine published by Butterick to sell its paper patterns, until 1883, but clearly the style existed before then, since

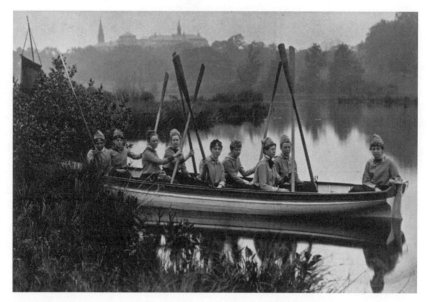

Crew of the *Argo,* 1879. Note the bloused shirts. Courtesy of Wellesley College Archives, photo by Seaver.

we see it here. *The Delineator's* winter catalogue (1888–89), in showing a ladies' yachting blouse, informs us that the style was "first published in June, 1883." In the catalogue for autumn (1889), four pattern illustrations for sports blouses appear: two sailor blouses, another nautical-style blouse, and a "tennis shirt."[1] Two have the corsetted silhouette of high fashion, but the other two are the baggy, unfitted "blouse shirt," as *The Delineator* calls them. It is these "sport blouses" that form the basis of the outfits that I focus on in this chapter—the crew uniforms at Wellesley from the 1870s to 1892.

The outfit was unusual for its time in that it was decidedly different from the fashionable look of those tightly corseted and bustled years. It seems to have appeared in response to need. In the photographs, it stands out for its originality. I can find no specific references to it anywhere, no explanations other than what follows in this chapter for its appearance and the date when it was introduced. If it resembles anything else from the time, it is the sailor suit of little boys, except paired here with a skirt instead of the knee-length stovepipe pants boy children wore. It was used for crew at Wellesley as early as the late 1870s, just a few years after Welles-

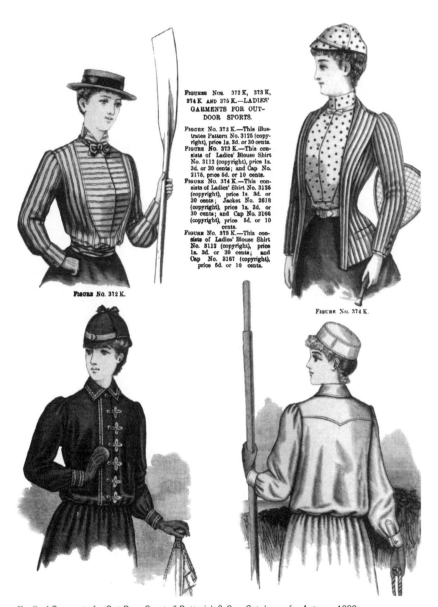

FIGURES NOS. 372 K, 373 K, 374 K AND 375 K.—LADIES' GARMENTS FOR OUT-DOOR SPORTS.

FIGURE No. 372 K.—This illustrates Pattern No. 3125 (copyright), price 1s. 3d. or 30 cents.

FIGURE No. 373 K.—This consists of Ladies' Blouse Shirt No. 3112 (copyright), price 1s. 3d. or 30 cents; and Cap No. 2175, price 5d. or 10 cents.

FIGURE No. 374 K.—This consists of Ladies' Shirt No. 3125 (copyright), price 1s. 3d. or 30 cents; Jacket No. 2618 (copyright), price 1s. 3d. or 30 cents; and Cap No. 3166 (copyright), price 5d. or 10 cents.

FIGURE No. 375 K.—This consists of Ladies' Blouse Shirt No. 3112 (copyright), price 1s. 3d. or 30 cents; and Cap No. 3167 (copyright), price 5d. or 10 cents.

FIGURE No. 372 K.

FIGURE No. 374 K.

"Ladies' Garments for Out-Door Sports," Butterick & Co., *Catalogue for Autumn*, 1889.

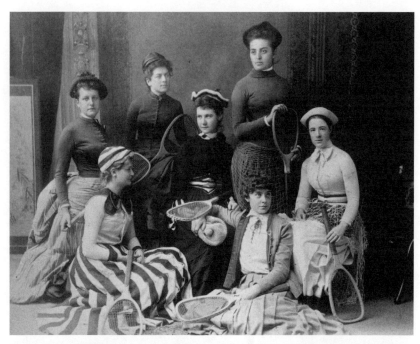

Wellesley College tennis players, Spring 1887. The two women center front wear loose bloused tops that contrast sharply with the tight basque bodices of the others. Note particularly the girl at the lower right: she forecasts the twentieth century—bare-headed, though clutching her tam, loose-sleeved, easy and relaxed—and the only one of the seven who does not wear a corset. Courtesy of Wellesley College Archives.

ley opened. It appeared at approximately the same time at Mount Holyoke, not for crew but for other outdoor activities. Clearly, it was an outfit for exercise, a gymnastic dress. It deserves mention here because it plays a twofold role. First, if it was a skirted dress with no trousers underneath, it sits somewhat precariously between the fashionable dress worn for sporting activities outdoors at the time and the truly athletic dress with trousers that women devised for gymnastic exercise indoors. Even though its loose top reflected Lewis's dictum, it really is neither one nor the other. Or it may have had trousers hidden underneath (see Cornelia Clapp's instructions for making a gymnastic suit in chapter 10). From this distance in time, we have no way of knowing for sure. Second, it provides the missing link that carries Lewis's unconfining baggy-topped dress into the twentieth century, to the new idea of sportswear. So the question is, why this dress, and why at Wellesley?

Wellesley College was founded by Henry Fowle Durant, a wealthy Boston lawyer turned evangelist, who, with his wife, wanted to build a memorial to their two dead children. Durant was a man of his time. He expressed his evangelical spirit in more than purely religious ways: he put great faith in the benefits of good health, believing it one of "five great essentials for a higher education for womanhood." Speaking at the new college in 1877, he declared: "Our war-cry here is the old proverb, *Mens sana in corpore sano.* We seek freedom from the physical chains which enslave women." Furthermore, he believed that health was not just desirable but a religious duty. "Trample in the dust forever," he thundered, "the old loathesome ideal of the gushing story paper and silly novel, with the baby face and the small waist and the small brain and the small sentimentalism. . . . Shake off those poisonous, false ideas which make girls destroy health for show, and be reformers and preachers of the new evangel of health."[2] To help the college do just that, he had found an idyllic country location fifteen miles from Boston on the shores of Lake Waban, a retreat for the wealthy from the heat of the summer.[3] The campus still retains its idyllic setting, reflecting Durant's careful attention to location over a hundred years later. It is regarded by many as the most beautiful campus in America. From the very beginning, Wellesley encouraged students "to row on the lake, to take long brisk walks, and to exercise in the gymnasium."[4]

To get the girls out on the lake, Durant supplied the school with three boats. Their broad, heavy mass ensured the safety of the rowers. Christened the *Mayflower*, the *Argo*, and the *Evangeline* (after a visit to the college by Henry W. Longfellow), these cumbersome floating structures could hold six to ten people at a time.[5] They were known familiarly as "the tubs." The girls sat side by side, each pulling on her own oar, usually in groups of eight with a coxswain.[6] The earliest extant photograph is from 1879, the end of the fourth year the school was in operation.

Rowing at Wellesley started as pastime exercise but proved popular enough that the school purchased more boats. The girls would float around on Lake Waban in the early evening, singing while they rowed, their voices serenading those on the shore. Thus, both rowing and singing ability became the necessary skills for the early crews, but as everyone agreed, what mattered most was that the girls sing well and be attractive. Athleticism and the strength needed to row well were not primary considerations in the

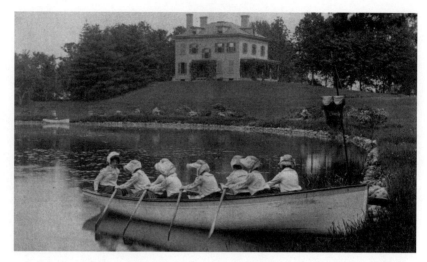

Crew of the *Evangeline*, one of the "tubs," 1884. Courtesy of Wellesley College Archives, photo by Seaver.

early years. Each year, the rowing activity culminated in Float Day (or Night), which led to a tradition at the college that lasted until 1948. A major annual event, it drew spectators from far and wide, with a special train bringing Bostonians to the campus as many as six or seven thousand at a time.[7] All visitors were invited personally, with hand-signed tickets to prevent the gate-crashing that proved to be a problem on occasion.

Because the event became a sort of theatrical presentation, a concert on the water, it was essential that the girls wear good-looking clothes. Each of the three upper classes had its own crew, with its own individual uniform and colors to distinguish one class from the others. These outfits, inspired and planned by the students themselves, changed with every entering freshman class but became formalized in the sophomore year when a class crew was chosen. They were attractive, sometimes nautical in style, loose and comfortable, and startlingly different from fashion wear. The anticipation prior to the unveiling of the sophomore suit, planned and executed in secrecy each year, built suspense and excitement. After its initiation, the sophomore uniform continued to be worn throughout junior and senior years until graduation— three years in all. The number of freshman crews, sometimes as many as nine a year, depended on the number of boats left. They, too, concocted their own costumes, but these, especially in the early years, were sometimes less

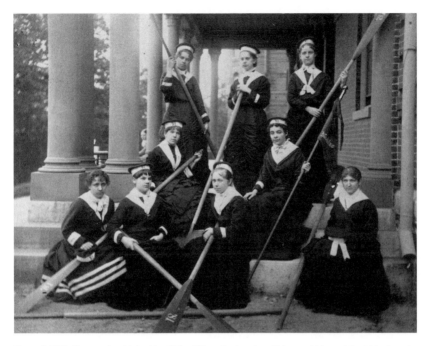

Crew of 1881. Hats, each with its identifying '81 on the band, and blouse shirts match, skirts do not. Courtesy of Wellesley College Archives.

impressive, less complete, and very likely less expensive than the upperclassmen's. They would consist of the same tops and hats, for example, but different skirts (depending on each girl's wardrobe), which barely showed below the gunwales of the boat when the wearer was seated to row.

By the first decade of the twentieth century, Float Day had taken on the character of a pageant, with all the participants' costumes following a single theme. The tradition finally died, a casualty of World War II austerity and a run of bad weather in the immediate postwar years. By the time it might have been revived, no one was left who remembered the character of the tradition.[8]

Of all the institutions of higher learning that began to educate women in the United States in the mid-nineteenth century, Wellesley was unique in having a rowing program from the very beginning. Attractive clothing played an important role from the start. I believe that these crew outfits are the earliest team uniforms for American collegiate women—possibly for any women in the United States—for a specific sport. In some measure following the fashion of their day, they form not only a record of the subtle changes in styles at the end of the nineteenth century but also a record of the increasing influence of physical education and its clothing on other activities, and of women's growing involvement and interest in the sport that became known as crew. These garments sharply point up the disparity, too, between fashion for sporting events out-of-doors and the sensible and comfortable clothing used for indoor exercise, hovering as they did between the two.

So what did the crew uniform at Wellesley look like? Anyone who has seen Dio Lewis's gymnastics dress will recognize its origins. It consisted of, in 1880s parlance, a "blouse," meaning any blouson-style, loose-fitted top that draped over the waistband or onto the hip. As fashion, it was approved more for children than for adult women.[9] It was, however, a style encouraged at that time by advocates of physical education for gymnasium dresses. From the 1860s to the 1890s, all descriptions of the gymnastic dress stressed the need for enough material in the waist, or bodice, to provide room to move the arms and upper body; for example, in this 1885 description: "The waist is quite loose, and long enough under the arms to enable the wearer to thrust the arms directly up without drawing upon the waist and belt at all. There should be plenty of room across the chest. . . . The sleeve is what is commonly known as a shirt sleeve, being perfectly straight. . . . It is prettiest when finished with a deep turned-over cuff. . . . A sailor or any large collar is used."[10] Just the kind of top a girl needed to pull those oars. To judge from this description and the pictures, it was the gymnastic dress that provided the model for the crew outfits in the early years at Wellesley. The difference lay in the lower half of the suit. Whereas the gymnastic dress was shortened to mid-calf, with Turkish trousers worn underneath, the crew suit had a full-length skirt and no trousers. After all, this outfit was worn in public, where men could see it. The attractive *Prydwen* crew wore the blouse costume in 1883, as did the crew of the *Evangeline*, manfully laboring to beach their boat even though virtually hidden under bulky sunbonnets in June 1884, and so did the crew of the class of '86.

The differences in the uniforms lay not in the style of the blouse waists but in the colors, the collars, the decoration, and the hats. The colors ranged from mid-tone to pale, but also with heavy emphasis on nautical navy; the collars were for the most part spread or, to use nineteenth-century termi-

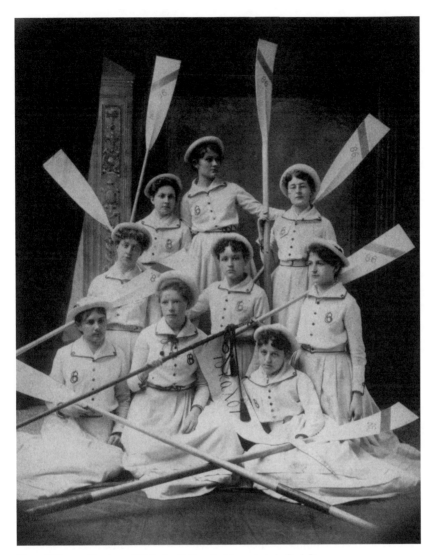

Class of '86 crew. Courtesy of Wellesley College Archives, photo by Pach Bros.

nology, "rolling collars"; the decoration depended on braid patterns and contrasting buttons, even, as in the class of '86 uniform, in the subtle positioning of the pockets. In the team photo, four members have pockets with a graphic "86" on the right breast and five have them on the left, a concession to the pairing of rowers on the boat's wide seats. The embroidered pocket would be on the side most visible to the spectators. It was the hats, though, that set the character of each crew. Ranging from an early coolie hat in the 1870s to a cap somewhere between a French Canadian toque and a Revolutionary Phrygian cap, they seem to struggle for appropriateness, not always succeeding. Perhaps the least appropriate from a sports point of view was the neck-swathing sunbonnet, and the most was the small rolled-brim sailor's hat of the class of '86. An amusing if incongruous though certainly status-conscious hat adopted by the senior crew of 1885, identifying them at a glance, was an adaptation of the mortarboard. Their dress, incidentally, was very plain, with a shirt-like top (not as bloused as in the previous years) and a straight, full, softly-pleated and gathered short skirt, falling just to the ankle—very unlike the fashionable ideal of the time.

The mid-1880s seem to have been a turning point in the orientation of the crew costume. With these years we see the same ambivalence already noted in outdoor sports clothing. Fashion generally prevailed, but a few holdouts opted for comfort. The gymnastic dress–inspired outfits of the early 1880s fell out of favor, to be replaced by much more fashionable outfits, however impractical they were. Their clearly corsetted, tight basque bodices topped elaborately swathed bustle skirts. Photographs show the overlap of old and new over a couple of years' time. The most graphically symbolic is of the class of '87 crew in their boat, facing to the right, countered by the "Specials" rowing in the opposite direction.[11] The "Specials" wear the sport blouse costume topped by a Rough Rider–sort of hat while the '87s wear their dark, form-fitting, height-of-fashion basque outfits, distinguished by light militaristic horizontal stripes accenting the front panel. Only their hats, dashing and sporty, echo those of the "Specials." Several other pictures of individual teams, all dating from these years, show the two separate styles coexisting: both the seniors (who trimmed theirs with elegant scrolled embroidery) and the "Specials" of 1888 opted for comfort and agility, with their bloused shirts and gathered skirts, while the junior crew of '89 preferred fashionable elegance, choosing long, torso-conforming jerseys draped at the hip with a bustled polonaise over a broad-striped, bi-colored, box-pleated skirt. The freshman crew of '91 perhaps best exemplify the equivocation of those years: they wore the blouse top but paired it with a straight, swagged, ungathered skirt, very probably bustled in back.

The first appearance of the jersey top in 1887 reflects an awareness not just of current fashion but of fashion for sport. It was similar in style to

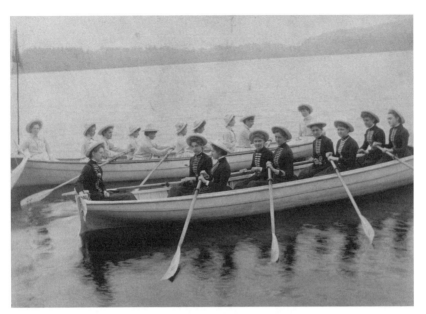

The Specials and Class of '87 crew. Note the corsetted basque bodices and the ensuing straight backs of the Class of '87, foreground, contrasting with the bloused tops and easier postures of the Specials behind them. Courtesy of Wellesley College Archives.

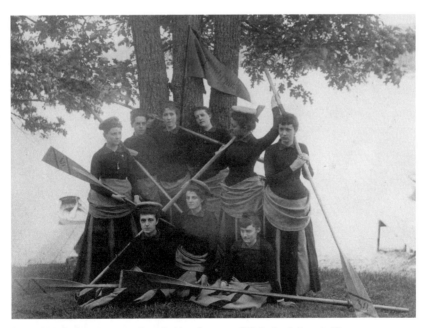

Class of '89 Senior crew succumbs to fashion. Courtesy of Wellesley College Archives, photo by Partridge.

men's athletic jerseys, mostly worn for baseball at that time, with its laced placket-front opening and small spreading collar; the idea was very likely borrowed from brothers at nearby schools.[12] A writeup of Float Day the following year mentions the Specials' "striking costume of broad blue and white striped, pleated skirt, [and] blue jersey with rolling collar."[13] Another style entering at this time was the turtleneck, already worn by male athletes but only then beginning to be adopted by women. None of the accounts name it as such, however; it was generally referred to as part of regulation gymnasium costume. Not for another five years would the term "sweater" be commonplace in the writeups of Float.

Two *Wellesley (Mass.) Courant* articles on the 1889 Float Day provide a wealth of information about the event and the costumes that year. The first, written for the May 24 issue by Clara T. Barker, Wellesley '89, displays a critical bent befitting a senior (and, indeed, makes one wonder whether she had some personal axe to grind). Her disgruntled report informs us that the class crews were still being chosen "more for their ability to sing and to be ornamental than useful." "Here . . . we have no races," she added, so "singing is a thing to be considered." But she didn't think it should be considered very much: "Strength should be taken into account also. Those girls should be chosen who are strong, muscular and energetic; girls who exercise for exercise's sake and not because they must; girls who have life and vitality enough enough to undergo such a training as would enable them to row in good form; the singing and comeliness should be a secondary consideration." She sounds aggrieved, but hers turns out to be a prophetic voice.

The second article, dated June 21 of that year, describes Float Day itself. Here we get the first real glimpse of the color of the class suits, complete with reporting as judgmental as anything in the fashion press of the time. The junior crew's "heliotrope . . . trimmed with gold" was "not so effective as other suits, because of its darker shade, yet [was] the most strictly nautical, and in its double sense, 'ship-shape.' The banner [was] an artistic and beautiful one of rich heliotrope silk, embroidered in gold." The "Specials" followed the juniors "in a striking costume of broad blue and white striped, pleated skirt, blue jersey with rolling collar, and edged with stripes of blue and white, and blue and white jersey caps. The banner is of white satin and blue ribbon, embroidered with blue, bearing the name of the crew boat, *Undine*."[14]

Of the nine freshman crews who marched and rowed that day, three surviving photographs remain; they support the observation that "all the costumes were pretty and some particularly original." Stripes were popular during the last half of the 1880s, as borne out by the number of times they appear in the uniforms: blue and white, red and white, some even with matching blazers. Without a doubt, though, the most unusual was a crew who wore "a true Scotch costume throughout," complete with glengarry caps and, in at least one case, a cairngorm brooch holding the plaid at the shoulder. Attractive, but not exactly the perfect outfit for rowing. The wave of the future, in fact, appeared with the sophomores, who made their "*debut* with great success." Their costume was "a simple but noteworthy one. The pleated skirt and jersey [was] of dark green and in front, in the usual crew, uniform style, the jersey bears, in larger numbers of lighter green, '91. The caps are round and stiff, finished with a visor and with black cord." The 1890s bore out their vision towards simplicity, as we shall see.

Attractive as the crew members all may have been, their prowess at the oars that year left something to be desired. "Almost all of them rowed evenly and with a strong pull, though not with the speed which might secure the Mott-Haven cup, even were Wellesley to excel in all other games." (Clearly, in the view of the writer, such a thing was not remotely possible.) Even "the singing did not prove so successful as heretofore, both on account of the wind and of an unhappy choice of tunes. For such an occasion it would be wiser to choose a . . . simple, and especially, since the high notes sound much thinner on the water, a *low* air." Not all observers were so disenchanted: that was the year Chauncey Depew, a Republican senator from New York who had lost his party's nomination for the presidency, attended Float as an honorary junior.[15] He even wore the juniors' heliotrope and gold pin to identify his allegiance, and was overheard to exclaim, "How charming!"—letting those who were near know that "his heart was won for Wellesley."

In more than one article on Float Day hints of something other than pure delight had started appearing by this time. Indeed, the forthright commentary of the period highlights the main weaknesses of the event, foreshadowing the changes that would occur in the following years. To understand better why these changes came about, some mention must be made of Lucille Eaton Hill and her influence on crew at Wellesley.

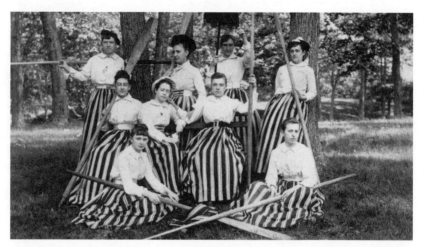

Freshman crew, wearing the popular stripes of the 1880s, 1889. Courtesy of Wellesley College Archives, photo by Partridge.

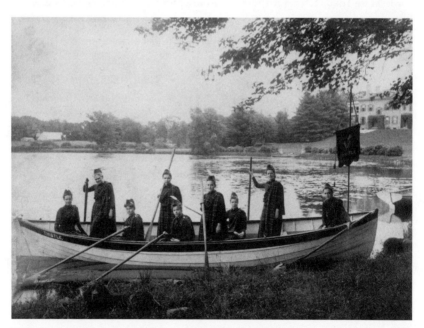

Miss Davidson's Freshman crew, resplendent in highland dress, 1889. Courtesy of Wellesley College Archives, photo by Partridge.

Until the time she arrived in 1882, "the boat crews at Wellesley were entirely in the hands of the students,"[16] and the tradition of rowing was well established. But there is no doubt that over the next twenty years she brought significant change. By the 1890s, she was training at least one hundred girls each year for crew. To prepare herself for the task—it must be remembered that no other program like this for women existed anywhere else in the country—she traveled to several men's colleges that offered crew, including Yale and Harvard, and learned everything they could teach her.[17] The earliest visible result of her research was in the introduction of spoon oars in 1883, used by the official class crews only. Freshmen and "Specials" still had to make do with the old-fashioned flat oars.

As the years went on, Hill trained her girls in a much more rigorous fashion, starting them as early as February indoors in the gymnasium on rowing machines. But since no racing was allowed at Wellesley, the advantage of the new design and training was moot. In this refusal to compete, Wellesley followed the pattern of the time at women's colleges, joining Mount Holyoke, Vassar, and Smith, which unanimously and strenuously discouraged any intercollegiate rivalry whatsoever, even though the question arose every now and then. They believed that the "sporting" element was masculine, rough, and unbecoming to young ladies.[18] Health and fitness were the raison d'être behind the programs in physical education, never competition. That was the official policy.[19] However, a *Boston Daily Globe* article of June 8, 1894, reported, "Racing was once the practice [at Wellesley], when the girls organized their crews at pleasure. But at the first of it one of the crew members was injured in an exciting race. This accident put an end to racing at Wellesley." Instead, the crews were trained to work together, maintaining form and dignity as they rowed gracefully over the lake. They would row in formation, creating stars and W's with their boats.

The 1880s saw an escalation in the emphasis on the costumes. Popular newspapers and magazines, fascinated by the new women's colleges generally, delighted in describing the outfits to their readers, probably stimulating even greater planning, time involvement, secrecy, and expense on the part of the sophomores. But by the 1890s, after at least a decade under Miss Hill's guidance, the program changed in several ways. The clothing simplified, paralleling what was happening in the gymnasium because of the introduction at that time of indoor sports. Furthermore, the 1890s saw the increased involvement of women in sports in general, with an accompany-ing fashion for fitness. Clara Barker's pointed remarks demanding more attention to athleticism and less to beauty were indicative of that new spirit.

Wellesley responded to the mood of the time, deciding "that the students were getting a one-sided development. There was too much brain work and too little physical strength developed to support the brain." The college took such "wonderful strides in the perfection of all its physical training, that its outdoor athletic work is now carried further than in any other college for women."[20] One result of this decision was to bring the best rowers from all classes together into an all-college team in 1891 to create the beginnings of a varsity crew. Eventually they became known as "the college eight." But the most influential change came the following year, when four new cedar shells, light and with sliding seats designed for crew, were purchased by the individual classes. These new boats brought not only a new quality of row-ing but also a seriousness of intent that had not been there before; by the next year, singing ability was no longer a requisite for crew.[21] Within two years, all the rowers at Wellesley were using the new boats.[22]

The sliding seats had one other significant effect. The voluminous skirts of the rowing uniforms did not allow the crews to perform well. Thus, in 1893 they devised a solution: they wore their gymnasium turkish trousers instead of their skirts to row. At Float Day that year the rowers appeared as usual, but as they approached their boats, they calmly removed their outer skirts and climbed in, ready for action. "The effect of this change, however, was scarcely perceptible from the bank," reported the Wellesley College magazine, *Legenda*, "and most on-lookers were unaware that it had taken place."[23] A photograph exists of the class of '94 crew rowing their sleek new boat, dressed in turtlenecked sweaters and, barely visible but dis-cernible nonetheless, bloomers instead of skirts. By 1895 the *Boston Herald* was moved to comment, one imagines with some regret, that "the costumes had not the variety of some years."[24] Although the attractive uniforms lasted throughout the decade, for the 1897 Float Day the *Herald* reported: "The class of '99 is the first to take the lead in abolishing the expensive crew suit, a relic of the days when the crew girls were chosen for their pretty faces and good voices and rowed in the college tubs. They wore, therefore, the regulation gymnasium suit, with white jerseys bearing their class numeral in green. Their caps were black, with green band, embroi-

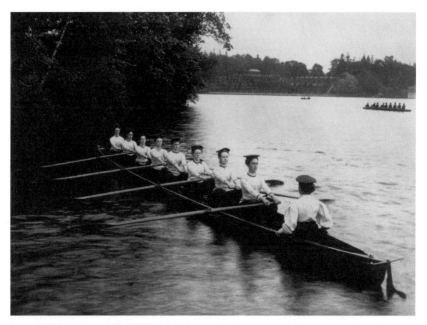

Class of '95 Freshman crew, 1892. Not only the new boats were streamlined, so were the uniforms by 1892. Courtesy of Wellesley College Archives, photo by Pach Bros.

dered with the name of the boat, Narcissus." All three freshman crews went hatless, another first. Miss Hill "was heard to say that 'they were the best freshman crew that had ever appeared on the lake.'"[25] In 1898 the clothing was not even mentioned in the newspaper accounts, and by the turn of the century, all the teams were wearing the regulation gym trousers and turtleneck or laced-front sweater.

The outfits of the mid-1890s had reflected the balloon sleeves and tailor-mades that were high fashion then. But sport overtook fashion, and function won the day. It is significant that the clothing finally adopted for this particular outdoor sport was a version of the gym suit, the first loose and bifurcated garment acceptable for women—and, it may be added, the earliest example of the comfortable clothing that eventually developed into what we now consider sportswear. Crew uniforms evolved from the loose gymnastic dress of the 1870s; then an ever-increasing awareness of fashion led to constriction; finally, the pendulum swung back again to the gymnasium outfit

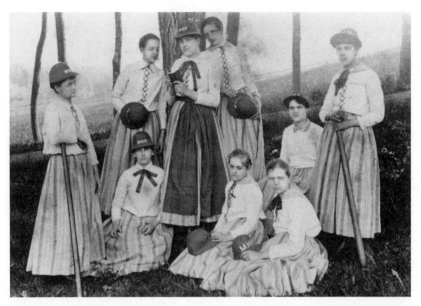

The Mount Holyoke Nines, about 1886. The uniform for baseball at Mount Holyoke echoes the crew blouse and skirt at Wellesley. Courtesy of Mount Holyoke College Special Collections and Archive.

of the day. They represent the earliest continuous use of uniforms for a single sport worn by collegiate women in the United States. Mount Holyoke College students had formed a baseball team sometime around 1886 or 1887 (and, interestingly, wore a costume, complete with laced jersey sport top and striped skirt, very similar to the crew outfits at Wellesley in those same years).[26] Other colleges also formed baseball teams for women at that time, quite likely also adopting a simple gathered skirt and loose top. As early as the 1860s, Vassar had designed its own gymnastic dress in gray with red trim, but it was used for exercise in the gymnasium only, not as a sport uniform.

That the outfits for rowing were successful may be seen in their use for other activities. Photographs depict girls in other settings wearing their crew suits, recognizable from the rest of the clothing worn in the pictures because of the hats, decoration, and very different, looser silhouette, usually based on the bloused top. The photograph of tennis players in spring 1887 is a good example. Of the seven young ladies, five are encased in the tight, bustled fashion of the day (two are even draped in polonaises made of tennis nets), but the two in front wear their crew uniforms. The one seated at the left wears her striped-skirted suit, so popular in the 1880s, while the other wears the laced-front jersey under her jacket. Only the one on the right is uncorseted, unlike the fashionable rest. The look of this clothing is startlingly modern, in sharp contrast to the 1880s signature look of the others. One is struck by its acceptance until one remembers that to row in a class crew was a mark of achievement at Wellesley. Thus, to wear this functional clothing was a mark of status on campus.

If Wellesley was the first school for women to use a common outfit for a single sport, it was the students themselves who generated the idea, thus laying the foundations of team uniforms for women.[27] One is amused at the detail and volume of the early outfits, even as one is amazed that the activity could be performed at all. Even if the thread of common sense in designing a blouse top with room in the sleeves, shoulders, and ribcage prevailed through the excesses of tight sleeves and bodices in the 1880s, one is sobered by the realization that it took twenty years to arrive at a uniform that allowed the rowers to do their job well.

THE DEBUT OF
THE
Gym Suit

OUT OF THE ENDURING INTEREST IN GYMNASTICS AND SPORTS CAME THE inevitable need for leaner, more sensible clothing for women who wanted to participate. While the Dio Lewis costume described in chapter 8 remained a staple for over a quarter of a century, it bowed to greater pressure when "boring" calisthenics finally gave way to challenging and competitive team sports, mainly in women's colleges in the 1890s. The first indoor team sport for women, basketball, devised by Senda Berenson at Smith College and based on the men's game, demanded a newer kind of clothing, a uniform style of dress that became known as the gym suit. This gym suit revolutionized women's clothing and set the stage for the easy clothing of the twentieth century that became known as sportswear.

There is scarcely a woman over the age of forty who does not remember with aching clarity just what her gym suit was like. My own, typical for its time and place in 1950s southern Ontario, was a shapeless blue cotton bag with a camp shirt top buttoned down the front with white plastic buttons and drawn in at the waist with an overlapping belt anchored by two more white buttons side by side. In my high school, athletic girls (the tomboys) demonstrated their independence by doubling the belt around at the back through the belt keepers and buttoning it there. The suit looked even worse this way than with the belt defining the waist. White, splotchy winter legs emerged from the romper legs, whose elastic got looser as the years wore on. Until we warmed up, goose-bump arms, with each hair standing straight on end in the cold gym at the beginning of every class, dangled from depressing, styleless short sleeves. (In fairness, I confess I do recall two girls in all my high school years who managed, with their long slender legs, slim, shapely bodies, and golden skin, to make even these look good.)

Each limp, dull, unironed suit was adorned with the wearer's name, painstakingly embroidered in white on the back. It was a task we were all assigned as we entered high school. If we were handy with a needle, we did it ourselves; if not, our mothers came to the rescue. Not only did this hone our needlework skills, but it also instantly identified each one of us for our teacher to single out should we fail to perform to her satisfaction. In the changing room after each class, we'd roll up the grungy, sweaty blue mass, wrap it around our gym shoes and socks, then stuff them into the bottom of our hallway locker, to forget about until the next gym class. Only the initial odoriferous gust on opening the locker between times reminded us of its existence. Rarely did we take it home for washing unless we were scheduled for inspection. Then the whole unsavory mess would go into the washing machine together.

Interestingly, although we girls all wore this same regulation gym suit, our teachers had nifty little sleeveless skirted tunics that gently skimmed their bodies, worn over crisp white shirts that perfectly matched the V-cut of the tunic neckline. Their gym shoes were spotless white, a bright extension of the trim ankle socks above them. Never did we question the unfairness of this.[1]

High school girls from the middle years of the twentieth century also remember their gym suit's particular color. Mine is forever imprinted on my mind as "gym suit blue," but other women from other parts of North America have reported green, gold, and even lavender. Some have actually insisted that they liked their version of the suit. Most of us, though, remember its style, its smell, and the mortification we suffered if the boys saw us in it because it made even the best of us look so awful. Whatever our reactions, the gym suit for North American women remains indelibly etched in our group memory. We all wore it, many of us hated it, and the rest, at a distance of some thirty to fifty years, still confess to a certain ambivalence. But oddly, in my experience over the past twenty years, more women today laugh and reminisce about this particular item of apparel than any other. It is a common bond we all, as educated women, share. And it represented a huge leap forward for women and their clothing. It was the first outfit designed for use within a socially accepted setting which allowed freedom of movement, comfort, and practicality. And, though limited to the confines of physical education, it was designed for sport.

The development of a regulation gymnastic dress began, as we have seen, with Dio Lewis, who not only generated an enthusiastic new interest in exercise but dictated the guidelines for suitable clothing for it as well. And as Mabel Lee, a leading educator in women's physical education in the United States in the first half of the twentieth century, noted: "It was the private woman's college that led the way in the establishment of physical education for girls and women in America. Physical activity class work had been offered at Mount Holyoke as early as 1837, at Rockford College by 1849, at Vassar by 1868, and at Smith and Wellesley College by 1875."[2] Certainly the impetus had grown out of the seminary movement, as we saw in chapter 8, but with the increasing interest in and awareness of the need to educate women equally to men, the visibility of the new institutions and their pioneering founders, teachers, and students grew too. So it is to the schools of higher education for women in the second half of the nineteenth century that we turn now to find the origins of the loose, practical, afashionable dress that eventually became known as the gym suit.

A few schools in particular give a fairly clear picture of the original approaches of the women's colleges to physical education. Mount Holyoke is foremost because it is the oldest continuously operating institution of higher education for women, and because Mary Lyon, as we have seen, insisted on exercise from the beginning. It also became the model that many other schools emulated as they opened throughout the country.[3] Smith College, younger than Mount Holyoke, is unique for introducing women's basketball. Others, such as Vassar and Wellesley, had their own personalities and their own solutions, so are invaluable as well.

To show just how far from the norm the women's colleges were in their approach, however, it is helpful to take a brief look at a large coeducational institution in North America: the University of Toronto, which opened in 1827 and accepted its first women in 1884.[4] Its yearbook, *Torontonensis*, was first published in 1898. Two years later a photograph captioned "The Gymnasium" showed a man in exercise garb, wearing tights and a form-fitting, short-sleeved pullover, rather like a leotard of today.[5] Throughout the next few years, men were photographed in team uniforms or, as with the "Gymnasium" man, in exercise clothes. Women, though, were consistently depicted in street wear plus academic gowns in all the yearbook photos. Not once was a women's athletics-related group shown in any kind of athletic dress, even though these were the years when the rigid rules of gender-driven propriety were beginning to slacken. In fact, the absence of any pictures of women participants would lead one to believe that women simply never indulged in any kind of sports. This was not the case. A piece in the 1903 *Torontonensis* on the women's athletics program of Victoria College[6] gives some insight into the true state of affairs: "Physical culture, too, is not neglected but is a department well patronized and much appreciated. Undoubtedly the most popular sport, however, is skating, which every girl seems to look upon as a daily physical necessity." A note in the same article mentions that the girls' hockey club (in Canada, hockey is, without further definition, ice hockey) had been formed the year before. Another note, in subdued tones, this one from the University College Women's Athletics program, perhaps reveals the reasons why the girls enjoyed skating so much, for in all likelihood, no other option had existed up to that time: "In 1901, a small and unassuming gymnasium was granted by the Senate [for women]."[7] One questions whether the men's gymnasiums would have been thus described, or, in fact, if the women's gym was even constructed after it was "granted."

It is possible that what drove the style of presentation in the yearbook photographs was the same set of conventions we observed in Part One: what was acceptable for women when accompanied by men was quite different from what was acceptable for women alone. And after all, the university world was part of the fashionable world since it was coeducational. Even so, it is clear that by the turn of the century, some attention was being given to women's athletics. The women's colleges, however, provide a very different picture. Let us return, then, to Mount Holyoke Seminary, and to Dio Lewis's influence there.

As noted earlier, Mary Lyon's calisthenics disappeared in the wave of Lewis's "new gymnastics" in 1862. Hers had been regarded as too much like dance by the pious evangelicals of the time, who shunned all such frivolities. Accordingly, wands, dumbbells, and Indian clubs swung in patterns took the place of the old-fashioned calisthenics, and helped the rhythm of new exercises. The outfit for the new exercises followed Lewis's suggestion—"a very short skirt with 'zouave' trousers drawn up just below the knee and falling over nearly to the ankle."[8] This was the first accepted outfit for women's gymnastic activity in a collegiate setting. It established the model for the future, with subtle changes that echoed the evolution of fashion over the next couple of decades. The style was not uniform, and as late as the 1890s, it is clear that the dresses were home-made.

Mount Holyoke's catalogue from 1864–65 warned students that they must provide "suitable clothing for the season and the climate, such as flannels, woollen hose, thick shoes, overshoes and an umbrella, also a dress suitable for gymnastic practice." The choice of style lay with the wearer. Over a decade later, in 1878–79, the only change in this directive was the addition of "leggins . . . and a dress for gymnastic exercises." The first catalogue to specify what this dress should look like appeared in 1882–83, when the description read, "The gymnastic dress may be of flannel (dark blue is preferred), made with a blouse-waist, sleeves full, belt loose, and the hem of the skirt seven inches from the floor."[9] That same year, 1883, gymnastics instructor Cornelia Clapp (who was also the zoology instructor)[10] wrote a *Manual of Gymnastics*, in which she finally gave clear directions to any dressmaker for creating the appropriate gymnasium dress:

> The dress may be of [wool] flannel (dark blue is preferred), made with blouse-waist, loose belt, sleeves moderately full, good length and closed at the wrist.
>
> It requires about 8 yards of flannel, single width, or four and a half double width, for the dress, including drawers, which may be pieced at the top with cambric.
>
> The dress should not be trimmed heavily; a flounce about six inches deep should be stitched on to the lower edge of the skirt, not put on the skirt, and a band of trimming to match collar and cuffs, or rows of braid, may be placed above the flounce.
>
> Width of skirt about two and one fourths yards, and seven inches from the floor.

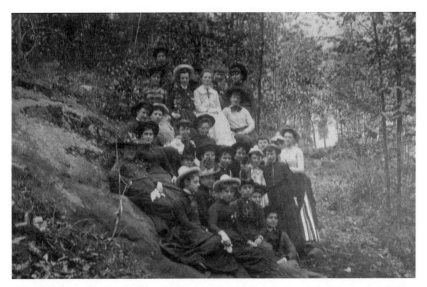

Mount Holyoke College students on an outing on Mount Tom, 1880s. Gymnasium dress mandated by Cornelia Clapp, similar to the crew outfits at Wellesley during the same period. Courtesy of Mount Holyoke College Special Collections and Archive.

> The waist should be made long enough under the arms to allow the arms to be stretched upward to their utmost extent without drawing upon the belt at all. Shoulder seam should be short, and arm-holes large.

Her final directive was: "Corsets and high-heeled boots are out of place in the gymnasium."[11] Clapp's description of the gymnastic dress comes to life in a photograph of students climbing Mount Tom in the 1880s, and in the crew uniforms at Wellesley at the same time. Interestingly, Clapp specifically mentions drawers as part of the outfit (even if "pieced at the top with cambric," a cotton), but never, in any of the photographs from either Wellesley or Mount Holyoke, do these show.[12]

The adoption of Dio Lewis's gymnastic system in the 1860s proved a critical impetus behind building a gymnasium at Mount Holyoke—no small feat in wartime. After a fund drive led by the governor of Massachusetts, who visited the school and was impressed by the gymnastic display put on by the students, it opened in 1865.

Vassar College took a slightly different approach, as it did to much else in the establishment of private degree-granting women's institutions in the

United States. Its first catalogue (1865–66) pointed out that the building housing the riding hall and gymnasium was still being built, but that "classes for Physical Training were organized and instructed in the corridors of the college by Elizabeth M. Powell." These corridors were "beautifully lighted, aired and warmed . . . [to] afford ample means of indoor exercise in inclement weather." Other "feminine sports and games" would "diversify the physical exercises," including "boating in the summer and skating in the winter, without danger of outside intrusion . . . archery, croquet (or Ladies' cricket), graces, shuttlecock, etc." A suitable dress was deemed "indispensable." Accordingly, "a uniform [was] adopted for the calisthenic classes in the College, the material for which can be procured and made up on arrival. . . . Every student will be required to provide herself with a light and easy-fitting dress, to be worn during these athletic exercises. It will be left optional with her, whether to wear it or not at other times."[13] The suit was referred to as a "simple uniform of gray and red sash." To judge from the illustrations, it too was based on Dio Lewis's gymnastic dress. But because it was mandated that all students wear the same dress, in the same material, this was the first uniform for women in a collegiate setting, or almost certainly any other, for athletic activity in the United States. Incidentally, Vassar is unique in even suggesting that students might wear their gym dresses anywhere outside of physical training. Generally, such freedom was prohibited. Perhaps the physical isolation of the college and its buildings from the town of Poughkeepsie had something to do with the leniency.

It is doubtful that the Vassar suit lasted long. Dr. Eliza M. Moser, who went to Vassar as resident physician in 1883, recalled in an after-dinner speech in 1920 that she had presented a request that same year on behalf of the director of the gymnasium to replace "the monotonous calisthenic exercises in very proper ankle-length skirts [clearly not the gray and red Turkish trouser outfits of the 1860s] by the newly developed Sargent system of gymnastics, physical measurements and divided skirts." She further reported that "an old faculty member" declared, "The girls will not stand for it," while another flatly stated, "They will not wear divided skirts."[14] Both proved to be wrong; the girls did, and willingly.

Although the women's colleges led the way in advocating exercise for women, the entire health and exercise movement was at its peak in these years. So strong was the demand for gymnastic dresses generally that popular magazines such as *Godey's*, *Peterson's*, and *The Delineator* all published articles on them, with pictures, telling how to make them, from the 1860s into the 1880s.

By the late 1880s, outfits consisting of full Turkish trousers and a "blouse" had taken precedence over skirted gymnastic dresses. One writer referred to "the fluffy little skirt" that "turned out to be no skirt at all. It is two skirts, a divided skirt, it clothes each leg separately. It makes a pretty drapery while the gymnast is motionless, but it does not interfere with the perfect freedom of the limbs. She is wearing Turkish trousers, after a model of the gymnasts' own."[15] In 1888 the dress reformer, Annie Jenness Miller recommended in an article, "Exercise for Women," "a regular costume . . . which will not impede or interfere with the free movements of any member of the body." It should "properly consist of a pair of full Turkish trousers with a jersey underwaist or blouse, which can be worn with an abbreviated tunic drapery [hard to visualize from a twenty-first-century perspective], if one be supersensitive to appearing in the simple trousers and blouse, which are now worn as the regulation costume in all of the popular gymnasiums patronized by both sexes."[16] Finally, in 1893 Butterick came out with a pattern for the gymnasium bloomer.[17] This coincided with the earliest manufacture of the garments by commercial companies, which heralded a new uniformity.

The question arises, then: Why was there a need for uniformity?

With the single exception of Vassar College, the gym bloomer as a uniform emerged because women began to participate in team sports, indoors, in the gymnasium.[18] Basketball was the first. It had been devised as a game for men by Canadian-born James Naismith at Springfield (Massachusetts) Training School (later College), in 1891. The next year, after its rules had been published in the *Journal of Physical Education*, Senda Berenson, who taught gymnastics just a few miles north at Smith College in Northampton, adapted it for women. She too published the rules of her game. Up until this time, exercise had meant calisthenics: swinging Indian clubs, waving wands, even Dio Lewis's "new gymnastics," which were a form of calisthenics. It was frankly boring. By contrast, this new, energetic game put vigor into the physical education program. It was snapped up by schools

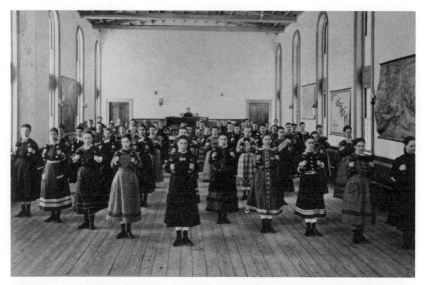

Calisthenics class, clutching dumbbells at Mount Holyoke Female Seminary, 1876. The dresses, no two alike, follow an updated 1870s version of Dio Lewis's preferred outfit. Only one girl, second on the far right, gives any hint of trousers under her skirt. Courtesy of Mount Holyoke College Special Collections and Archive.

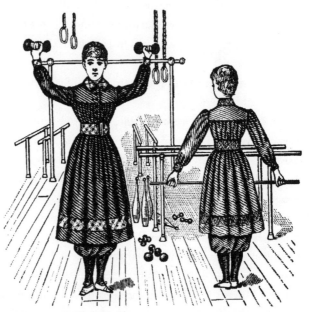

Calisthenic suit, "dark green and Scotch plaid serge," 1890. The immediate precursor to the skirtless suit devised for basketball. *The Delineator*, July 1890, 65.

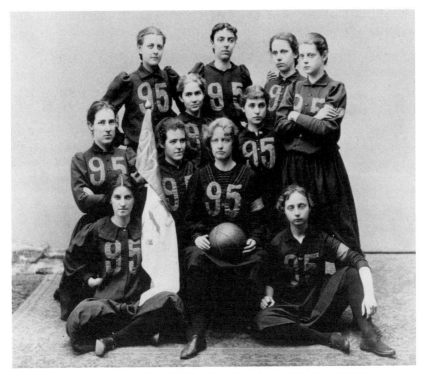

Smith College basketball team, class of '95. Note that the outits vary in design, and that the numbers haphazardly cover details of the suits. Courtesy of Smith College Archives.

everywhere in an amazingly brief period of time: by 1894 or 1895, most schools that had women students had basketball for women. In many cases it was not part of any regular physical education curriculum; often it was introduced through women's athletic associations or the efforts of the girls themselves.[19] Under whatever auspices, this game spelled the end of the old skirted gymnastic dress. It was simply too bulky. With the skirt finally banished from the gymnasium, the bloomers shortened and widened to give the appearance of a short skirt, and the blouse was buttoned onto the bloomer waistband. That much women gained. What they sacrificed was the ability to wear this new garment out-of-doors, where someone—specifically men—might see them.[20]

At first, we see variety in the styles of the outfit, even on the same team. They all seem to be based on the gymnastic dress pattern that *The Delineator* offered as early as September 1891 or the variations on the sailor blouse that began turning up in the 1880s for sports and yachting. The sailor collar seems to have been preferred, but even with variations in style, all of the blouses were paired with baggy bloomers of the Zouave type that hung past the knee. By the mid-1890s, uniformity in design began emerging, and by the early years of the new century, a uniform as we think of it had taken shape. This suit, with slight variations, was worn by all girls participating in all athletic endeavors indoors. In outdoor activity, only when the field was remote and hidden from the public could the girls wear their gym suits, and even then, they had to cover their legs with skirts while going to and from the playing fields. Trousered legs for women simply were not accepted—not even when the trousers looked like skirts.

A notable, and for the time shocking, exception was in California. (California's reputation for leading innovations in education certainly applies to the area of women's clothing for physical education, as we shall see again later.) In his history of Stanford University, Orrin Leslie Elliott wrote, "Basketball, a very recent sport, was taken up with enthusiasm and in 1894 an off-campus game was played with the Castilleja School in Palo Alto, Stanford losing 13 to 14." This event stretched the mores of the time as far as they could go. "This is the initiation of public athletics for the girls here," one of the juniors wrote. "They played in their gym suits on the grounds by Castilleja Hall. They rode to the game in a bus in their suits just as the men do. While some are quite opposed to such doings, there seems to be very little said in the matter. I don't feel in the least like entering into any such thing, nor do I feel like criticizing the girls who do, if they keep on their own ground or play with the prep school girls."[21]

Two years later, however, girls from Stanford and the University of California played a sensational game in the San Francisco Armory. (Interestingly, basketball at this time was only a women's sport in the West.) At California's insistence, and much to Stanford's scorn, only women were permitted in as spectators.[22] In this, the girls from Berkeley followed the tradition of modesty already established at Smith College in Massachusetts.[23] Not only were men banned from seeing women striving to win, but they were prevented as well from seeing them in public wearing trousers. Stanford won, by a score of 2 to 1. With a ball that did not bounce but was passed from player to player, the game was slower than it became later, and scores were lower. These two games were the very first interscholastic ath-

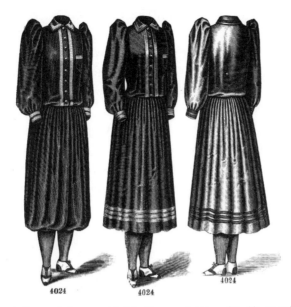

"Ladies' Gymnastic Costume": "may consist of the blouse and skirt or of the blouse and trousers, as preferred; but it should be understood that the trousers and skirt are not to be worn together." *The Delineator*, September 1891.

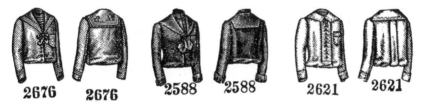

"Misses' Sailor Blouses and Tennis Shirt." Butterick & Co., *Catalogue for Autumn*, 1889, 16.

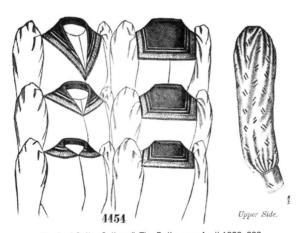

"Ladies' Sailor Collars." *The Delineator*, April 1892, 333.

letic contests for women. The eastern schools categorically refused any such recognition of competitive spirit on the grounds that it was unladylike.

Basketball was not the only team sport women played. Within eight years of basketball's appearance, the game of field hockey was imported from England by Constance Applebee, a visiting scholar at a Harvard Summer School program in athletic training, first opened to women in 1896. She came to the wilds of New England in the summer of 1901 bearing her hockey sticks, eager to teach the new game to collegiate women.[24] Obviously, this was a game that had to be played outdoors, so what to wear? The *Boston Sunday Herald* later reported:

> When hockey was first introduced to Smith . . . the question of the proper costume immediately arose. Many of the girls thought they must wear bloomers, instead of skirts, in order to play well, but Miss Berenson said:
>
> "Well, girls, since we have to do all our running after we leave college in skirts, isn't it wise to learn to do it gracefully?"
>
> That settled it, and now the girls think that skirts are best, after all, because they often catch the ball when it would otherwise go out of bounds. Besides, they do not want to ape their brothers, or to be athletic in any sense such as men give the word.[25]

Whatever Miss Berenson's reasons, the truth behind the choice lay more in the conventions of the day: the sport was played out-of-doors, so skirts had to be worn. It was as simple as that. The players all wore roughly the same long skirts and tops but differentiated their teams through hats: one side wore tams, the other sailors. The one concession to all the running the game required was that the skirts were "short," that is, some four to six inches off the ground. It is interesting to note that this tradition was maintained when the game was revived as an intercollegiate sport for women in the late 1970s. The correct uniform remains the skirt in the form of a short kilt, still worn today. But the seeds of that kilt lie in the mores of turn-of-the-century America.

From the beginning, then, outdoor team sports for women, whether crew at Wellesley from the 1870s, baseball at Mount Holyoke in the 1880s, or field hockey at Smith, devised different styles of uniforms—skirted ones—from those trousered styles worn indoors, in the gymnasium. This dichotomy persisted until the 1970s.

The gym suit that emerged with basketball was a two-piece, inky blue-black serge, a tightly woven, rather harsh and hard-wearing wool, not too thick, but dense and scratchy.[26] The entire suit was made out of this material. The bloomers were really almost two full skirts, pleated to confine the bulk of material, and gathered at the knee. The crotch rested at knee height, often cut in a single large gusset, up to eighteen inches square, and set in on a diamond pattern. These were usually called "divided skirts," but as we have seen, the terms "bloomers" and "Zouaves" were acceptable too. The "blouse," or "waist," was similar to the one described earlier, dating from some ten or fifteen years before, which allowed the arms to move freely in all directions and which buttoned onto the bloomer's waistband. The women wore long black cotton stockings, held in place under the bloomer with garters, and flat rubber-soled shoes. The whole outfit in the mid-1890s cost under six dollars including the shoes.[27]

Interestingly, almost everyone, no matter where she lived, wore this same outfit, even in the humid, warm South. No regional differences in climate had any bearing on the approved—and hot—garment. I believe that the reasons for this were twofold. First, all the early instructors of gymnastics were trained in only a handful of schools, mainly in Massachusetts and New York. These women carried their programs far and wide throughout the country, but primarily into the Midwest and the South, even into Canada, and as they went, they took their regulation gym costume with them. Second, as industry production took over, supplying first universities and colleges, then high schools, with the garments for physical education programs, a limited number of choices existed. And the companies seem to have been located in the Boston area. Only California schools (the University of California, Stanford) used suppliers located in the West.[28]

A few gymnastic directors attempted to design different gymnasium costumes, notably at the University of Michigan and Stanford. Dr. Eliza M. Moser, a medical doctor (Michigan, 1875), returned to Michigan in 1896 as dean of women and professor of hygiene (not an unusual combination of credentials at that time). She had also graduated from the Anderson Nor-

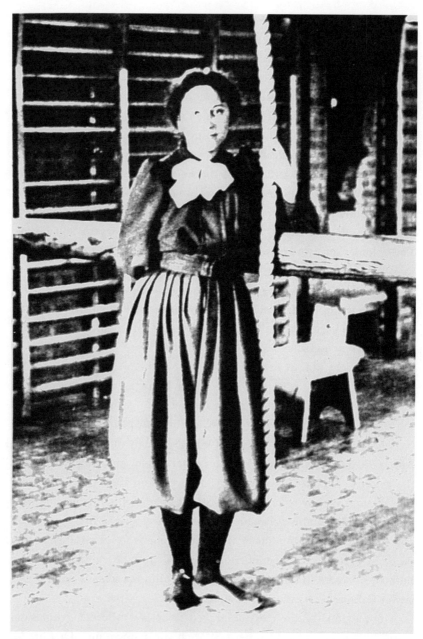
Senda Berenson wearing the new basketball uniform, about 1893. Courtesy of Smith College Archives.

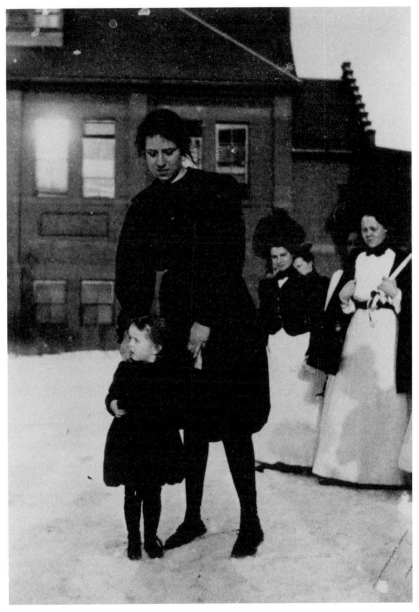

Basketball player and mascot wearing the serge gym suit, about 1901. The observers in the background wear the fashion of the day, in sharp contrast to the look of the clothing for sport. Courtesy of Smith College Archives.

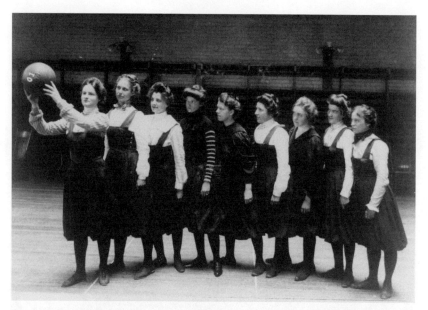

Eliza M. Moser's gymnasium uniform, worn by the Michigan basketball team, 1896. Courtesy of Bentley Historical Library, University of Michigan.

mal School of physical education in New Haven and had studied at the Sargent School of gymnastics in Cambridge, Massachusetts. It was she who had gone to Vassar as physician in residence in 1883 and wanted to change the program and dress for gymnasium work at that school. When she came to Michigan, she designed a uniform to be used there. Called "the most novel thing about the whole programme" by the *Detroit Free Press*, it consisted of the typical serge bloomer, but rather than buttoning onto a blouse top, it attached instead to a

> low-cut bodice of the German peasant pattern with narrow bands
> passing over the shoulders. This bodice buttons under the left arm and
> fits the figure closely, giving the exact lines of the body from the arm
> pit to hip. It never pulls or shifts with any motion of the body, the
> arms and shoulders being left perfectly free. Under the bodice will be
> worn a sweater or jersey of peculiar design with full sleeves to the
> elbow leaving the forearm uncovered. This suit leaves the outlines of

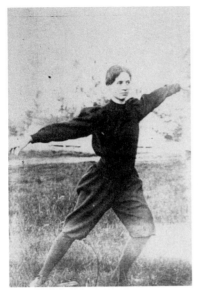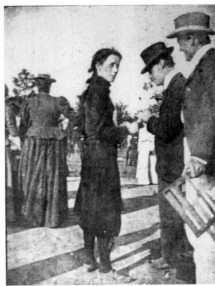

"The Stanford Gymnasium Suit" and the Berkeley version, both about 1896, unique at the time for the narrow knicker bottom. Courtesy of University Archives, The Bancroft Library, University of California, Berkeley.

the neck, shoulders and back fully revealed to the instructor who can thus catch at a glance any defects in the pupil of figure or movement. The usual gymnasium stockings and shoes complete the outfit. The skirt and bodice will be dark blue, and the sweater or jersey yellow, making the suit a veritable university uniform.[29]

It remained in use at Michigan for at least a decade. Photographs indicate that a new model replaced it by about 1905.

Stanford and Berkeley also attempted different designs, but neither seemed to have even the small success the Michigan suit enjoyed. The "Stanford Gymnasium Suit" appeared in photographs sometime after 1896,[30] the year of the famous Stanford-Berkeley game. Possessing a feminine, dressmaker look, it featured the narrow, unpleated knicker bottoms similar to those men wore at the time, but, in a surprising departure from the gym suit norm, the waistline sat at the small of the back, dropping in front to curve beneath the belly. The top appeared to button up the front, and probably buttoned onto the knickers as well. A high-cut funnel neckline set into a deep curved yoke finished the bloused bodice. Berkeley's suit, however—recorded in only one photograph—was perhaps the most startling for the period. The young woman wearing it, her posture relaxed and more expressive of the twenty-first century than the 1890s, appears to be almost in a time warp, with her knicker bottom and her simple, unadorned top that lacked the fussier details of the Stanford suit. We today can recognize her as one of us. Apparently, though, it was too avant-garde for even the daring Californians to wear; it appeared nowhere else, vanishing completely, to be superseded by standard gymnasium suits.

If the ideal gymnasium suit presented something of a problem for athletic women at the time, so did the underwear to wear with it. Few sources refer to it at all. We do get a glimmer of what was expected, however, in the third annual catalogue (1894–95) from the State Normal and Industrial School, later renamed the Women's College of the University of North Carolina, still later the University of North Carolina at Greensboro. It stated that the "gymnasium outfit, including a pair of gymnasium shoes, *a union undersuit* [my emphasis] and an over suit of blue serge, is required to be of uniform material and make, and cannot be made at home."[31] This represents the only reference to underclothing in connection with gymnasium dress I found in any of the institutions I visited, and one of the few directives that indicated how the emergence of uniform style in the suit came to be.

A major exception to the norm appeared in a series of articles in 1910 and 1911 by "A Non-professional Observer, Leonhard Felix Fuld, LL. M., PH. D." These three articles dealing with reform of women's dress for exercise were published in the *American Physical Education Review.* They discussed, among other aspects of the gym suit, the underwear worn with it ("if the student wears underwear, as should always be insisted upon . . .)."[32] It is clear that the author is addressing his remarks to teachers of physical exercise at the high school level; nevertheless, many of his comments are more universal. His caustic articles ridicule the programs as well as the outfits girls and women wore for them. He was not alone for his time in attacking the "physical torture of a waistband cutting into [the] abdominal walls" caused by the multiple layers of cloth in the overlapping waistbands, but he was the most outspoken:

By actual count it has been found that this costume has nine thicknesses of material at the waist. The serge bloomers have three thicknesses of material, lining and stiffening; there is a separate belt of two
thicknesses of lining to button the blouse to the bloomers; there is a
belt on the blouse consisting of two thicknesses of lining and the
blouse itself with its folds of material adds to the thickness of this
mass of material at the waist. In addition the underclothing worn by
the student may add three additional thicknesses of material to the
waist line and in some cases even more. The student accordingly
wears twelve thicknesses of material at the waist.[33]

Fuld was the only writer I found who expressed concern about the gaping of the various parts of the gymnasium suit—at the waist, where it buttoned; at the side, where the bloomers fastened; and at the
knee—commenting on "the mental disquietude resulting from the fact
that the wearer is "always coming apart at the belt" when engaged in vigorous exercise. "No refined woman," he warned, "can enjoy herself in the
gymnasium when this nagging consciousness is constantly present."[34] He
also was the only one who addressed "mental discomforts" and

the injurious effects of round elastic garters—little bands of torture
worn around the knee as bracelets worn around the wrist—they permit their pupils to wear them in the gymnasium because they are the
most convenient. It is true that when removed at the end of the gymnasium lesson they leave deep-cut furrows, but it is claimed that when
they are worn the stockings present a prettier because more taut
appearance. . . .

The mental torture which the student suffers from the existing
conditions at her knee results from the fact that with the activity in
the gymnasium there seems to be constant danger of exposure at the
knee. Much of this danger is fancied rather than real. Yet to a sensitive girl or woman this consciousness is a perfectly real discomfort.
Ordinary thrift and tidiness on the part of the student would seem to
be able to remedy this condition by the renewal of the elastic band at

the knee of the bloomers as frequently as may be necessary . . . [otherwise] there is always a likelihood that during exercise the leg of the bloomers will ride upwards and leave a portion of the leg exposed.

He recommended instead of the round garters ("an instrument of torture worthy of the Middle Ages") "a stocking or garter girdle with garters at the sides which do not exert any pressure over the bladder," one that crosses "the sacrum in the back and slants down just on top of the trochanter, buckling over the pubic bones." He warned that the novice might at first fear that the girdle would slip down, but assured his readers that this would not be the case, and that they would be "delighted" with its lack of interference.[35]

In addition, Fuld blasted the "present day gymnastic costume for women" as "outrageously unhygienic," adding: "In explanation of this statement it should be borne in mind that gymnasium costumes are almost invariably made of non-washable material,—usually of coarse, scratchy serge, or heating, moisture-absorbing flannel. Furthermore, the students seldom wear any underwear while exercising. In this way all of the perspiration and other skin exudations from the surface of the body are absorbed by the gymnasium suit which itself is never washed."[36] By "underwear" one assumes that he was speaking of a union suit, rather than a chemise and/or drawers—but perhaps not.

The general unwashability of the gym suit, and the problems that led to, seem to have been universal. By the time Fuld was writing his diatribes, a movement was under way to find a solution to those and other difficulties identified by wearers. Florence Bolton, director of the women's gymnasium at Stanford, had previously complained that a suit might be worn for "years without cleansing; the blouse especially is charged with oil and perspiration. Where a sweater replaces the blouse, its name is fully suggestive of its condition." She too criticized the existing suit for its mass of cloth binding the waist—up to four bands—but unlike Fuld, she lay the blame in a startlingly feminist fashion:

It produces what someone has spoken of as the "over-sexed" figure with abnormal protuberances above and below. These belts, usually fairly snug to begin with, are actually tight in many positions. . . . Men are undoubtedly somewhat responsible, directly or indirectly, for many of the absurdities in women's dress. Necessarily without experience in the matters upon which they pass judgment, often without any physiological, economic, artistic or other basis, their dictates are entirely arbitrary, but they dictate nonetheless. They love a certain tailor-made conformity. They allowed women to go into gymnastics with the understanding that they should not make themselves look too dreadful and unfeminine.[37]

Her solution was to design a suit that had no waist at all. Based on the English gymnasium slip, a knee-length, sleeveless, square-necked tunic with a straight yoke holding box pleats front and back, hers incorporated the English top with the American bottom, or bloomer.[38] It fell loose from the high yoke, and was lightly "girdled" rather than belted. Underneath, the gymnast wore a "washable guimpe," or shirt, adding to its hygienic appeal. Fuld sang the praises of this new outfit:

> Her costume consists of a one-piece slip which has no belt and no waist. A girdle loose enough to rise and fall and to return to place in the various positions assumed by the student in the gymnasium, is fastened firmly across the back and drops low in front, fastening with a snap. There is no pressure and as the suit is in one piece there is no danger of exposure or of coming apart at the waist. There is no sailor collar to flap in a most disconcerting manner about the head and ears of the student while she is in an inverted or semi-inverted position. The gymnasium suit is a one-piece slip which comes over the shoulders with two shoulder straps. At the neck a guimpe of some thin, soft, washable material is worn in place of the heating and irritating flannel, or the hard, scratchy serge.[39]

The only problem with this suit, as he saw it, was the reluctance of students to wear an outfit with no waistline in that very waist-conscious period.[40] For whatever reason, this outfit too found little outside acceptance, although it was adopted by the University of Wisconsin and possibly others, and was used to some extent into the 1920s. It remained in use at Stan-

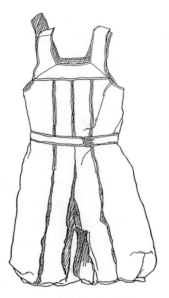

The suit patterned after the English gym slip worn at Stanford and the University of Wisconsin into the 1920s. Drawing by the author from a suit in the Stanford Archives (AM-79–12.13) donated by an alumna, Class of '29.

ford throughout the 1920s. For costume historians, however, it is remarkable in that it was a very early harbinger of the waistless fashions that were to sweep the world a decade or more later.

Possibly the major reason why the Bolton suit failed to capture a greater audience was the introduction, perhaps as early as 1908, of the middy. As we have seen, the sailor blouse and its variants had been commonplace for exercise since the 1880s, and sailor collars were the norm for the wool serge gym suits. Whereas the sailor style had been a true blouse, with its baggy waist drooping over the skirt or bloomer waistband, the new middy hung straight from shoulder to hip. Best of all, not only did it have cleaner lines, but it also was made of cotton duck. For the first time, then, the sailor blouse or middy had the benefit of being not just cooler but washable. Fuld wrote in 1910 that it had "come into use and into great popular favor" during the previous year; indeed, when there were no facilities for changing clothes, girls were encouraged to wear the top and a skirt over their bloomers so they might remove the skirt and be ready for exercise in little time.[41] Since the same voluminous serge bloomer was worn with it, one wonders at the bulk it must have produced under the skirts. Sometimes, for outdoor sports (where the players might be seen in public), it was worn with a "shortened" skirt. Another variation appearing at about the turn of

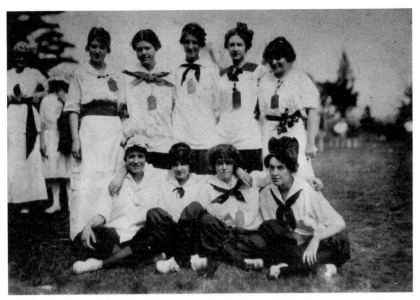

Middy blouses paired with baggy bloomers, about 1910–15. Compare the middy-wearers' silhouettes with the high-waisted fashionable dress in the background. Collection of author.

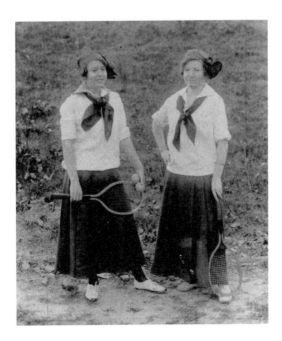

Champion tennis players wear the middy paired with a "short" skirt. Women's College of North Carolina, 1911. Courtesy of Photograph Collection, University Archives, Jackson Library, University of N.C. at Greensboro.

the century was a turtleneck pullover, borrowed from the men's schools, worn with the bloomer. But basically, the middy-and-bloomer combination was the gym suit used in high schools and colleges for the next twenty-five years, until it was finally abandoned about 1930.

Even the middy was not without its drawbacks. Once again, the critical eye of L. F. Fuld draws them to our attention. Ever alert to the "sensitive" nature of female students, he pointed to the low V neckline as a possible source of chill, although he admitted that "the danger of catching cold because of the low-cut neck [was] more apparent than real." His solution was to insist that a "chest guard provided with the blouse be worn." In addition: "When engaged in work on the heavy apparatus, the blouse frequently becomes disarranged [at the neckline] so as to expose the student's chest and breasts. This objection is also not entitled to much weight, since such exposure is not considered improper at a ball, or at the opera, and furthermore men are very seldom present in a gymnasium class." Far worse was what happened when "the student is in an inverted or semi-inverted position." This not only caused the "sailor collar to flap in a most disconcerting manner about the head and ears of the student," but brought even greater misery to the wearer because the blouse, "which has no waist, frequently rides up and in such cases exposes the trunk of the student in a manner which is likely to cause serious embarrassment to the student and places her in a condition in which she lacks that mental quietude so much to be desired in gymnasium work."[42]

Nevertheless, it was worn universally. A few minor changes were made by the 1920s: the bloomer might be a slimmer knicker, and the sleeves of the middy were sometimes short. This was the outfit our grandmothers or mothers wore in high school and in college. In fact, it became synonymous with "schoolgirl" in those decades. And it permitted girls to do things they had never been able to do before. They could run, play, leap, dive, hurdle, exert themselves. It cannot be stated too strongly that before gymnasium suits were devised, women were not permitted any of this activity, in large part because they were not permitted to wear the clothing that made it possible.

To cast a different light on the gym suit at this time, we should look at the clothing that male athletes were wearing. The late-nineteenth-century male gymnast wore an outfit not terribly unlike the figure-revealing tights and tops that American women wear today, only usually all black. Annette Kellerman, the famous Australian swimmer who in 1910 "designed her own swimming suit" (giving no credit to her inspiration), creating a scandal in the process, directly borrowed the outfit men had been wearing for gymnastics for at least a quarter of a century. It consisted of a form-fitting body covering with very short sleeves and a scooped neckline, and black tights.[43] While girls were modestly encased in yards of navy serge, boys were wearing knickers and short-sleeved pullover shirts. Even before the middy blouse was introduced, as early as the 1890s, men were wearing primitive versions of tank tops and shorts, all brief, all washable.

Much of the twentieth-century development of gym suits had to do with clothing design generally. It is not coincidental that street wear took on the waistless line of the middy after 1910. In fact, college athletic wear was as much as fifteen years in advance of fashion. The outdoor basketball uniform from Mount Holyoke College, with its knee-skimming pleated skirt, dates to 1910, and the waistless suit experiment and Fuld's despised round rubber garters eventually became symbols of the flapper in the 1920s. The gymnastic outfit had heralded an unconstraining kind of clothing for women long before the leading designers of the time, including Paul Poiret, who boasted of "abandoning the corset," and Coco Chanel, who "introduced" the idea of sporting sweaters based on English menswear. One might not have thought that the lowly gym suit, worn in the United States by what amounted to a handful of privileged young women, would ever make any kind of impact on fashion—indeed, would ever be seen at all in those circles. Gymnastics and sports, however, and the accompanying clothing became fashionable in their own right, and were written up in every major magazine for women, and even in general interest magazines such as *Harper's Weekly*. And these articles were illustrated. The proliferating image of the athletic American girl, so popular in the Gibson version, was a phenomenon of the period, a sort of pin-up of the time. Popular illustrators such as Harrison Fisher projected her as an ideal, and often portrayed her wearing, if not a gym suit per se, then a variation of it, with the turtleneck sweater and daring knee-length skirt that were worn for outdoor sports during the 1910s, long before short skirts were seen anywhere else. The correlation of athleticism and American beauty, tied to the new ideal

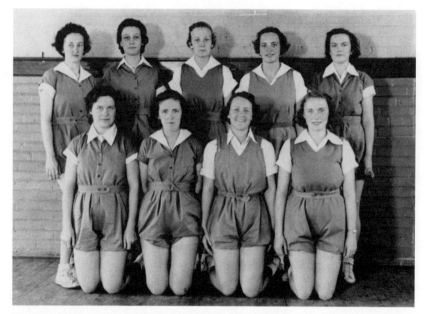

The washable cotton romper suit, from the 1930s. Courtesy of Photograph Collection, University Archives, Jackson Library, University of N.C. at Greensboro.

of the college girl, had a distinct influence on the fashions of the day—if not immediately, then subtly and over time.

By the 1920s, the gym suit seemed to flounder, as it sought a new form. The Stanford bloomer-jumper, of very lightweight wool, worn with a cotton blouse underneath, was one variation. Team uniforms took other directions: short tunics worn over shirts with knickers were one; shirts and shorts were another, appearing as early as 1929 at Rockford College. But the jumper idea seemed sensible, and in 1931 the accompanying bloomer shrank into a romper, with baggy elasticized legs that fell low on the thigh, generally just above the knee. It was worn either with or without a blouse. Unbelievable as it seems, this was the first completely washable gym suit ever designed.[44] It prevailed in many schools throughout the 1930s.

In 1933, however, Mildred Howard at Mount Holyoke College, working with the sporting goods company Wright & Ditson, started on the path to the design of the gym suit most of us remember with something between affection and horror. Her first attempt was a shirt and box-pleated shorts combination. The shorts hung straight, looking like a short skirt, and were flattering to most figures. These were soon discarded at Mount Holyoke, however, when Miss Howard realized that the girls preferred wearing the outfit with the shirttail out, hanging so low that the shorts vanished entirely. Her final design was based on the tennis dress. It had a romper as the base and a removable skirt that girls could wear over it if they wished. For certain activities such as gymnastics, the skirt generally remained off; for sports it generally stayed on.

In a letter written to Mildred Howard in 1947, Eleanor Edwards of Wright & Ditson, who had worked closely with Howard in creating the new style, credited her with the innovation.

> You were definitely responsible for the adaptation for gymnasium costumes, of the tennis dress which we are now using for the majority of the colleges we outfit. . . . And there is no reason in the world why you shouldn't claim that distinction!
>
> And Mount Holyoke was the first college in the East to adopt, for Physical Education classes, the *cotton* wash suit which is now so universally worn for gymnastic activities. And certainly no one can deny that for this purpose cotton is a great improvement over the wool materials! It was an important step forward—not only from the point of view of hygiene, but also from the standpoint of style—the bright colors of the cotton are so much more attractive than the drab navy and black of the wool materials.
>
> It is our sincere belief that these changes in gymnasium outfits must have done a great deal for Physical Education as a whole. Certainly they were bound to increase its popularity with the students, since they meant a girl could wear an attractive outfit that she liked—instead of a dreary (and often dirty!) suit she loathed, and hated to wear.[45]

With certain modifications, this gym suit became the symbol of physical education for girls from the 1940s through the 1960s, even as the middy and bloomer had been during the early part of the century. My own high school gym suit, with its camp shirt top, elastic-legged short bloomer bottom, and belt with two buttons at the front, was an ugly variation in a sharp blue that can only be described as unforgettable. Another variation used elsewhere was the skirted jumper with matching bloomers underneath. Although the move was slowly and inexorably toward a solely bifurcated garment, it took a long time to get rid of the skirt altogether.

Even as the romper-style tennis suit provided the basic model in mid-century America, one must note the exceptions. Schools in at least two states, California and Texas, chose to dress high school physical education classes in shirts and shorts as early as the 1940s. The shorts were navy blue cotton twill, the shirts either camp style or T-shirts. Once again, the wearer's name had to be embroidered (in navy) on the shirt pocket and down the white stripe of the shorts.[46]

One other new feature accepted by around 1930 or 1931 was short socks. Up until this time in America, women's bare legs simply were never seen in public, not even, up until the mid-1920s, for swimming and bathing. Women did not dare to venture onto a public beach without stockings. Indeed, in many cities they risked arrest for indecent exposure.[47] So the ankle socks worn with the romper-and-shirt gym suit of the 1930s completed the revolutionary look and allowed even greater freedom of movement and comfort.

The tennis-style gym suit came in many colors, blue being a popular choice, but others were an odd sort of sage green, yellow, lavender, and even red. Often, especially in the private schools, different colors signified the different classes, freshmen, sophs, and so on, recalling a tradition that harkened back to the crew uniforms at Wellesley and to the earliest days of team sports at Smith and elsewhere, when the numbers and trim on the navy serge collars and cuffs were in class colors.[48]

Eleanor Edwards's comments about attractiveness notwithstanding, the question of modesty had been an issue since the very beginning, as in the furor over wearing gym suits in public. Even the skirted gym suits of the 1940s, 1950s, and 1960s presented modesty problems. Although the bloomers matched, or were attached in some cases, women felt that letting them show was not respectable. After all, if they were under the skirt, they were underwear. This problem led to some interesting solutions. Girls tucked the skirts up into the legs of the bloomers to create, in effect, a second layer of bloomer. It has been suggested that this was to keep the skirts from falling in their faces as they did acrobatics. Possibly so. But having

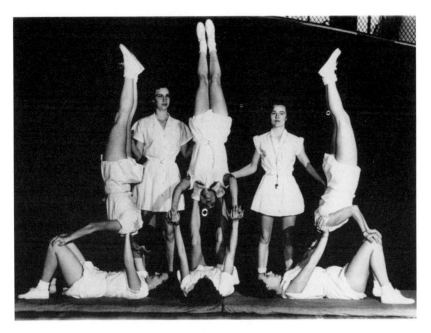

The tennis-style suit whose skirt could be tucked into the bloomers beneath when the situation called for it, 1950. Courtesy of Photograph Collection, University Archives, Jackson Library, University of N.C. at Greensboro.

undergarments show in those years, in any form at all, was simply no more acceptable than bare legs had been a generation earlier.

The gym suit persevered into the 1960s and even the 1970s in some areas of the country, especially in parochial and private schools, but finally died of natural causes sometime toward the end of that period.[49] In colleges, they vanished entirely, to be taken over by non-regulation shorts and T-shirts. But interestingly, in those years of turmoil, when women were beginning to come into their own in so many ways, women's athletics virtually vanished from college and university campuses. The decline had begun earlier, but it took hold in the 1960s. Over a ten-year period, in Big Ten yearbooks the only reported women's activity even remotely resembling sports was cheerleading. Of course, the big business of college sports for men really took off at that same time.

But beginning in 1975, a short while after the passage of Title IX, ensuring female students equal access to athletics, the yearbooks began to report on new intercollegiate teams for women: basketball, soccer, field hockey. And each sport had its own uniform. Basketball adapted the T-shirt and shorts, soccer much the same, and field hockey used the kilt, usually tartan. No one style of gym suit remains; uniforms for various activities have taken over. Specialization has found its way even into the gym. But the gym suit remains bound in memory, hated and loved, and little understood as to its significant role in twentieth-century America.

TAKING EXERCISE CLOTHES
TO
New Places

Women Biologists at Woods Hole

BY THE 1890S, THE SEEDS OF CHANGE IN WOMEN'S DRESS HAD BEEN planted. Inevitably, they came from outside the world of fashion. The dress reformers who elected to wear the "rational dress" at the Chicago Columbian Exposition in 1893 argued that the sight of many women attired in the revolutionary costumes would go far towards convincing a frankly skeptical nation that simplified clothing was preferable to the fashionwear of the day.[1] They readily admitted that the reform dress on single individuals would be "almost sure to be condemned as ugly at first sight," just as the original bloomers were, even as they argued that it wasn't any "intrinsic ugliness" that caused their downfall. Instead, they explained, it was "their oddity."[2] It is interesting to note that the Chicago fair and the introduction of women's basketball occurred in the same year. While dress reform as daily attire failed, the gym suit was just getting started. No doubt its success was the result of its specific application for wear in the gymnasium, for playing a game. There was no ambiguity about its usage: so it is to that usage we turn to see how clothing for sports achieved what decades of earnest reformers had failed to do.

The turn of the century must have been a heady time for young college women. Here they were, breaking from tradition, few in numbers but already the focus of the popular press as they sought higher education, already held up for comment, both positive and negative. Even those from

modest backgrounds stepped into the spotlight by virtue of their enroll-
ment in one of the colleges and universities mushrooming throughout the
country. Because the women who chose to be educated were extraordinary
for their day, and were, almost by definition, outside the mainstream, it is
not surprising that they, above all others, rapidly adopted the new clothing
for exercise. Indeed, they carried that clothing into the wider world.

A wonderful example of how that was accomplished may be found
among the pioneering women biologists who did their fieldwork at the
Marine Biological Laboratory at Woods Hole, Massachusetts. Their experiences demonstrate the struggles that women faced in achieving success as
scientists, hampered not only by society's expectations about their behavior
but also by the physical constraints of something as basic as their clothing
in a discipline that took them wading in the water. Through them, we see
how the new gym suits and bathing suits of the day began to fill the needs
of women whose lives were changing, who required more comfortable and
sensible clothing to do their work, and to do that work in public.

Gaining "marine experience" was a popular pastime of the Victorians.
Young ladies especially enjoyed observing the flora and fauna of the
seashore and recording what they found in their art. One such young lady
was Mrs. Alfred Gatty, who collected "and mounted seaweeds and sold
them to make a living." She published one or more books that she illustrated in color, using seaweed to create the images. The marine biologist
R. F. Scagel noted that women played a large role in British marine biology,
"and it is my understanding," he said, "that the science grew out of the art.
Some of these ladies making pretty pictures with seaweeds wanted to know
more about them and began studying them." Mrs. Gatty was one of the few
women—indeed, as far as I know, the *only* woman—to record her thoughts
about her clothing while on her collecting expeditions. So unusual and
compelling was her observation that Scagel included it as a preface to his
treatise on marine algae in British Columbia and northern Washington.
Gatty remarked in 1872:

> About this shore-hunting, . . . many difficulties are apt to arise; among
> the foremost of which must be mentioned the risk of cold and
> destruction of clothes. The best pair of boots will not stand salt water

many days—and the sea-weed collector who has to pick her way to save her boots will never be a loving disciple as long as she lives. It is both wasteful, uncomfortable, and dangerous to attempt sea-weed hunting in delicate boots. As for the hardier hunters who have learned to walk boldly into a pool if they suspect there is anything worth having in the middle of it, they will oil their boots. Next to boots comes the question of petticoats; and if anything could excuse a woman for imitating the costume of a man, it would be what she suffers as a sea-weed collector from those necessary draperies! But to make the most of a bad matter, let woollen be in the ascendant as much as possible; and let the petticoats never come below the ankle.[3]

Mrs. Gatty was an amateur, gathering specimens for her art. As such, even though her work had given her much knowledge and experience in the field of seashore collecting, she had no standing in the scientific community of her time. This situation was the norm. As we have seen, however, the last third of the nineteenth century was a period of new beginnings. So it was for women in science, and to tell their story in America, we turn once again to Mount Holyoke College (still Seminary then), to Cornelia Clapp. She arrived to teach at Mount Holyoke in 1872 and retired as head of zoology in 1916, having shaped the development of the discipline there and encouraged young women to study science throughout her long tenure. In 1874, barely a year after her arrival, she spent the summer at Louis Agassiz's Anderson School of Natural History at Penikese Island off Cape Cod.[4] Agassiz, one of the greatest scientists of his day, a teacher at Harvard and a founding father of American science, believed in the dictum "Study nature, not books." That summer, Clapp learned to collect marine organisms and study them from life. She and other colleagues who studied at Penikese brought that philosophy back to Mount Holyoke, where her department became well known into the late 1960s for its emphasis on the study of living (or recently living) animals.[5]

It was this same Cornelia Clapp who also taught gymnastics at Mount Holyoke throughout the 1870s and 1880s. Accordingly, it is not surprising to learn that her students, as one wrote to her parents in 1877, were sent out to collect "bugs and things" from the woods, streams, and fields surround-

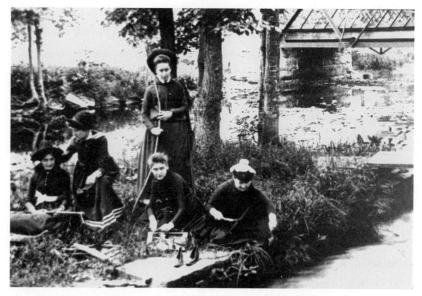

Mount Holyoke Female Seminary students collect and study specimens along the banks of Stoney Brook, about 1880. Courtesy of Mount Holyoke College Special Collections and Archive.

ing the campus. Nor is it a surprise to learn what they were wearing for that that activity, so unusual for girls of the day. The clothes were identical in style to the crew uniforms at Wellesley, made according to Clapp's guidelines, but they were worn both for outdoor exercise and collecting at Mount Holyoke. A photograph taken sometime in the 1880s, shows a group of students crouched beside Stoney Brook, the stream that flows through the campus. At first one might think they were picnicking, but a closer look reveals that the girl on the far left holds a net, and there are containers on the bank that could hold specimens. Rather than enjoying leisure time, these students were working, collecting organisms that lived in the water. The clothes—clearly matching, clearly uniforms—allowed them to do that with ease. They are all wearing the same baggy bloused tops and gathered skirts, even the same style of shade-giving hats that the Wellesley crews wore. A pair of rubbers sits on the rock beside them—the kind that the 1886 Bloomingdale's catalogue called "Ladies' Croquets," situating them firmly in the world of sports and outdoor games. They sold for forty-five cents a pair. Here they were meant to protect delicate feet from the wet bank of the stream if a girl pushed out too far with her dipping net. More than anything else in the photograph, these rubbers, laid out ready for use, clinch the argument that we are looking at a collecting expedition. It seems clear, then, that Clapp the biologist recognized the benefit of the comfortable, sensible clothing that she recommended as a gymnastics teacher, and had the imagination to extend its use beyond the confines of exercise.

Cornelia Clapp, an enthusiastic field biologist, studied with the greats of her time who were establishing the field. Interestingly, and following the pattern set by Mrs. Gatty and her ilk, much of the early aquatic scientific work in the Northeast was both done by and supported by women—as donors (such as the Women's Education Association of Boston), as students, and as investigators. Several unsuccessful attempts to establish marine teaching laboratories finally led, in 1888, to the founding of the Marine Biological Laboratory (MBL) at Woods Hole on Cape Cod, today an internationally known center for marine biology. Clapp was there every summer from the start. Indeed, when her work there inspired her to get her Ph.D., she took a leave of absence from Mount Holyoke to study at the newly founded (1890) University of Chicago. She completed her degree in 1896 at the age of forty-seven. Her own experience led her to encourage her colleagues at Mount Holyoke to complete doctorates as well, thus beginning the tradition of highly educated and trained women scientists that Mount Holyoke has been known for ever since.

She continued her affiliation with the MBL, returning every summer to Woods Hole to work first in the lab, then the library, and finally as a trustee until her death in 1934. But she wasn't the only woman there. Photographs reveal that there were many others. They also reveal the onerous conditions under which women had to work—conditions they perhaps never seriously questioned.

An 1895 photograph from the MBL archives tells the story. Of the twenty or so people in the picture, fourteen are women. Everybody is involved in digging, inspecting, collecting with nets, and all are working in and out of the water. A look at their clothing is edifying. The men wear hip boots, roll their pants above their knees and wade barefoot; at least one wears knickerbockers with soft shoes. This is the clothing of sport. Another kneels in the water, protected by his hip boots. They wear sweaters and shirts, some with their sleeves rolled up. But the women! Doing exactly the same work, they uniformly wear long skirts that have been shortened to

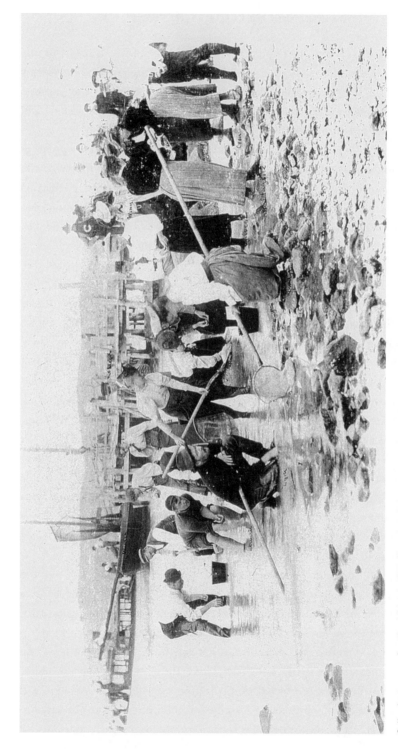

Collecting party at Cuttyhunk Island, 1895. Note that all the men wear practical clothing; the women do not. Courtesy of Marine Biological Laboratory Archives, photo by Baldwin Coolidge.

just above their ankles in an era when fashionable skirts invariably covered the foot. Deep, bunchy—and probably home-sewn—hems raise the skirts on the two women wearing lighter-colored skirts (probably wool, as Mrs. Gatty suggested). At least one of the others, very daring, has hiked her skirt up between her legs rather like a diaper and secured it through a ring device on the front, making it look as if she were wearing trousers. She is not. In a different but infinitely more customary convention, the woman using the dip net in the foreground bends her knees, keeping her straight back rigid, clear evidence of the inevitable corset. Of the fourteen women, only two are bare-headed.

From our vantage point, these women seem almost unbelievably constrained by their clothing. It is startling, then, to realize that all of them are wearing some version of what amounts to new and even reformed dress—the shirtmaker and skirt of the New Woman. The "New Woman," the social phenomenon of the 1890s, referred to women such as these: women seeking reform, women who worked, women who sought an education, women who needed sensible clothing that was relatively inexpensive and more easily laundered. Although menswear was being machine manufactured by this time, only select items of women's clothing were mass-produced: outerwear, underwear, and shirtwaist blouses. This last, combined with a flaring skirt, became the "uniform" of the period, much as jeans and T-shirts are in our own time. Many of the shirtwaists in this photograph are worn with men's-style ties in the fashion of the time. All of them have the full puffed sleeves of the 1890s. Not one woman has rolled her sleeves up, even though their hands must have been constantly in and out of the water. By contrast, none of the men wears a tie. Indeed, at least four men wear jerseys or sweaters, also relatively new inventions of the period, taken from the world of sports.

So the conventions of fashion bound women at this time, even though men showed them a different model. The only thing these women are wearing that bows to their practical needs (unlike the earlier Mrs. Gatty) is a good pair of boots, tight-fitting, mid-calf, and likely made of rubber. Rubber galoshes had been developed in the United States as early as the 1830s, but rubber boots (or wellingtons) weren't developed until 1885, after Mrs. Gatty's time. However, something called "Arctic overshoes," another American invention, had been in production as early as 1872, and incorporated a rubber galosh with a felt top. By the mid-1890s, then, these women could choose from a variety of footwear suitable for wading in the water, and in this photograph they clearly seem to be wearing them.[6]

Like people in every age and society, all these women were wearing clothing dictated by the social mores of their day. To do their work, they made slight adjustments, but not enough to unsettle the conventions of the period. Other photographs from the same time show women working in the lab at Woods Hole or relaxing after the day is over. All wear very conventional clothing; after all, they were working and socializing in mixed company. Thus the Mount Holyoke girls could wear their gym suits while gathering samples within the secluded confines of the campus, but even twenty years later, these same college-educated women did not have that freedom when they were interacting with their male colleagues on Cape Cod. Indeed, it would take another fifteen years before the clothing for sport could be adapted for work by the women biologists at Woods Hole.

A rare photograph of Ellen Swallow Richards, taken at Jamaica Pond outside Boston in 1901, bears this out.[7] Perhaps best known today as the founder of home economics, Richards was the state water analyst for Massachusetts and the first woman faculty member at MIT, in sanitary chemistry. Interested in the public health implications of water quality, she is shown here, accompanied by a man, gathering algae with what appears to be a small kitchen pot and a shallow kitchen ladle—suitable, one must agree, for the founder of home economics. To do this, she is wearing a dark, sober outfit, long skirt tucked around her feet, and a matching straw hat—all in the fashion of the day. As one of the leading women scientists of her time, she could have set a new standard of dress for the job if anyone could. But by the time this photograph was taken, she was an older woman, most likely firmly captured by her generation's conventions. Besides that, she was in a suburban setting with a man accompanying her, both conditions that would stifle any thought of adopting clothing more suitable for her work.

To judge by the photographs in the MBL archives, it wasn't for another decade, until 1909 or 1910, that women working with men finally wore innovative dress, the clothing for sport and exercise, as their dress of choice when collecting samples in the field. By that time, the phenomenon of girls playing team sports in college and wearing gym suits with bloomers had been folded into popular acceptance. The gym outfit, by now a combination

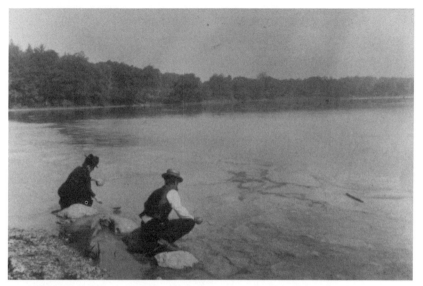

Ellen Swallow Richards collecting samples at Jamaica Pond, 1901. Courtesy of Sophia Smith Collection, Smith College.

of heavy black bloomers and the new hip-length white middy blouse with its black tie, was a great improvement. It was washable cotton, its long sleeves could be rolled to the elbow or it even could be short-sleeved, a real innovation. It was lighter in weight, perfect for warm weather and physical activity, and it was a huge success from the beginning. Based on the midshipman's uniform, long, waistless, and worn loose over the bloomers or skirt beneath, it became the uniform of the American schoolgirl, heralding a new silhouette that would remain the rage of fashion for the next fifteen years or more.

So what part did it play at the MBL? A photo from the summer of 1910 shows the women in middies, but still upholding the "skirt convention" as they tramp with male companions over the boulders of the rocky coast. That same year the women wore their bathing suits, cut on similar nautical lines, to collect. The next year, the women broke the skirt convention and wore either their bathing suits or their gym suits for collecting in the water. A few wear their middies with bloomers, while others wear a variety of bathing dresses, all covering the body in appropriately modest fashion. Of course, they still wore the long black stockings that never entirely went

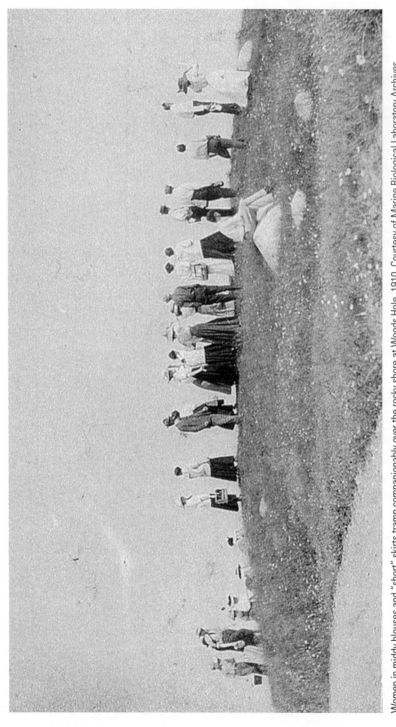

Women in middy blouses and "short" skirts tramp companionably over the rocky shore at Woods Hole, 1910. Courtesy of Marine Biological Laboratory Archives.

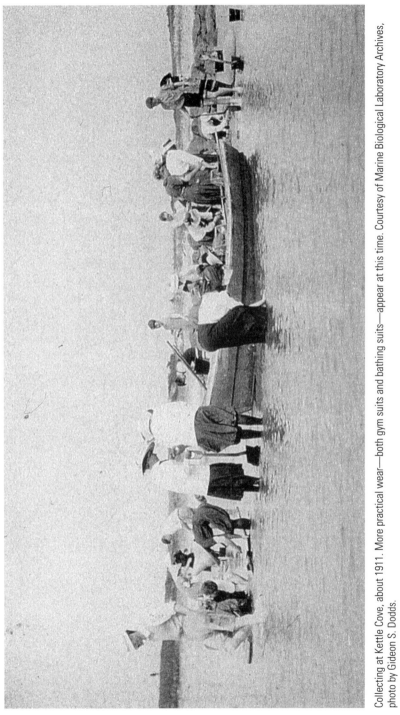

Collecting at Kettle Cove, about 1911. More practical wear—both gym suits and bathing suits—appear at this time. Courtesy of Marine Biological Laboratory Archives, photo by Gideon S. Dodds.

away until the mid-1920s, in contrast to the man striding through the water with his pant legs rolled up above his knees. One woman, however, seems oblivious to her long skirt dragging in the water—obviously a holdover from the earlier, more conventional times. So, finally, some fifteen years after the earliest photograph of researchers collecting, the women are free to bend, stretch, get wet, and enjoy a modicum of comfort because they have adopted the clothing they normally wore only for sport. The revolutionary middies were so welcome by this time that they were adopted for general summer wear. Two pictures from 1911 show two versions, one the standard white, the other dark. Both are worn by women on board collecting ships from the MBL. The short skirt and the white tennis shoes are both still worn a hundred years later—a testimony to the practicality of sporting clothes as they evolved in the early twentieth century.

A major factor here is that all these women were probably students or faculty from colleges and universities around the country. They were therefore used to seeing and wearing this unconventional type of dress, especially when away from the reach of urban proprieties. Once again, though, a picture of a social gathering at the MBL reminds us that sporting dress was limited strictly to non-social events. The clothing for both men and women is very different here: feminine dresses for the women and tailored suits for the men, even in the Cape Cod summer setting of the MBL. Although the transition to functional clothing was well under way for the aquatic biologists of the Northeast then, the conventions of polite society still held sway. Nevertheless, the clothing these women were used to for athletics and exercise in their universities had begun to transform their work, to facilitate the ease of collecting.

Those biologists were ahead of their time. In the 1920s and 1930s, trousers for women finally came into their own, first as knickers, then as slacks. As yet not fully accepted in all situations, both were worn only for leisure, away from the city. In 1924 Cornelia Clapp noted the effects of the new, relaxed fashions on South Hadley. "The old ladies on Park Street," she observed (she herself was seventy-five at the time), "have been scandalized by the appearance of *bare legs*—Girls and boys going to swim in the Upper Lake. They have not had the *advantages* of Woods Hole!"[8]

By the late 1930s the transformation was complete. In informal situations, neither bare legs nor trousers for women were cause for comment any

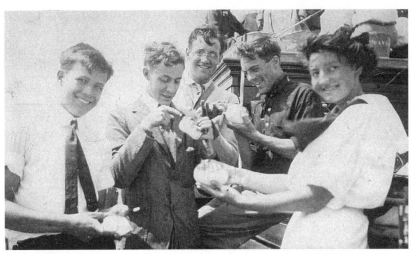

A woman aboard an MBL collecting ship wearing a standard version of the middy, about 1910. Courtesy of Marine Biological Laboratory Archives, photo by Gideon S. Dodds.

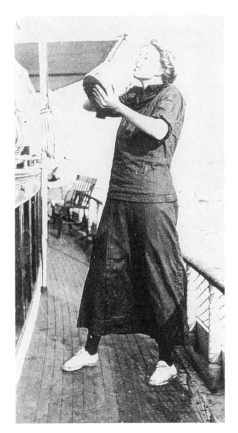

"'Frantic' takes a drink," about 1910, wearing a dark version of the middy with a matching skirt—clothes for sport. Courtesy of Marine Biological Laboratory Archives, photo by Gideon S. Dodds.

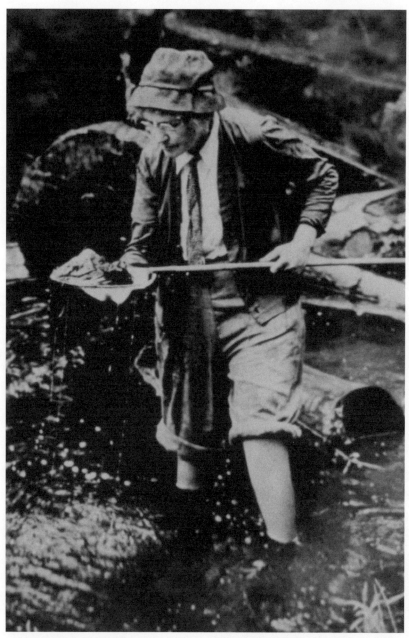

Ann Haven Morgan collecting in menswear, her customary choice, 1945. Courtesy of Mount Holyoke College Special Collections and Archive.

longer, especially on college campuses. Indeed, we see photographs of aquatic biology students at Mount Holyoke collecting in a stream, wearing hip boots, rolled chinos, denims, or bare legs, all in the casual American style based on the cut of men's clothing. The female instructor shown here, who had taken Clapp's place after her retirement in 1916, adopted male dress for her own personal style in the 1920s and never gave it up. Did she influence her students in their dress? Since no evidence exists, we can only guess. That adoption of male dress among a certain segment of women in the 1920s may have played a very significant role—one that hasn't been explored yet—in the acceptance of trousers for women. But this was a time when many new influences were changing the face of the nation, and indeed the world. The date of this picture is 1938, immediately prior to World War II. The clothing of the women aquatic biologists reflected the new role of sportswear in all walks of American life. Finally, women were dressed as casually, as personally, and as functionally as any man had been in the 1890s, forty years before.

THE MERGING OF
Public and Private

Sportswear and the American Style

THE WOMEN BIOLOGISTS AT WOODS HOLE CANNOT HAVE BEEN ALONE IN taking the physical education clothing they had worn as students out of the gymnasium and wearing it for activities that demanded more common sense than fashion in dress. The impetus that inspired them to adopt it for their collecting was likely the same one that made the middy-bloomer combination the uniform of schoolgirls everywhere by the late teens and 1920s: it was tough, hard-wearing, easy and comfortable, even if somewhat bulky. Further, it signified a certain youthful air, and a casual but reasonable rejection of the social proprieties that were still very much in operation at the time. It was entirely American, the first clothing for women that could be so identified since the American or bloomer costume of the 1850s. Unlike that short-lived attempt at reform, this one stuck: by the 1920s, the new outfit was entirely accepted. Although many presume that World War I provided a catalyst for change in women's dress at this time, in actuality the changes had been well under way years before the war began. The new outfits for exercise predated by over a decade the lean, pared-down fashion wear Chanel and Patou claimed to have introduced for sport. Whatever the timing, what is important to realize is that the inspiration behind the new clothing came, as we have seen, from American women's higher education, an area far removed from Paris fashion houses.

Clearly, the time had come to abandon the rigid patterns of the past and to look towards a new, modern approach to women's dress. The change was slow, and it depended on many converging factors in order to reeducate the taste and judgment of society. Participation in outdoor sports was the prime mover. If sport captured the imagination of America in the nineteenth century, it caught fire in the twentieth. The modern Olympic Games had a great deal to do with that, but so did the team sports of colleges and universities. For example, the football rivalry in the eastern schools, most notably in its beginnings between Princeton and Rutgers in 1867, then with "the Game" between Harvard and Yale, dating from 1875, grabbed the attention of the popular press. From then on, the press embraced its role as purveyor of sports heroics—and is still going strong in the twenty-first century.[1] These newspapers and magazines, illustrated with images of the players wearing their uniforms, introduced a new hero to the world. And once girls began to play, they too appeared in their appealing sports outfits. The burgeoning interest in sports of all kinds and the allure of life at elite schools as reported in the illustrated papers, brought it all to the public's eye, and provided the atmosphere needed to accept the new attitudes evident in the clothing designed for various sporting activities. Sports, then, almost unwittingly, accomplished what no amount of dress reform had been able to achieve in the previous century.

Hand in hand with the need for new types of clothing came innovations in textile and clothing manufacturing. It is often difficult to figure out which was the chicken and which the egg. However, alongside the introduction of football and other outdoor sports in the late nineteenth century, companies began to produce the knitted shirts, sweaters, and underwear that the players needed. One such company was Munsingwear, which opened in Minneapolis in 1886 and incorporated as the Northwest Knitting Company the following year to manufacture knit underwear for both men and women. Over the course of the next decades, the company provided knitwear for sports, and claimed to originate the classic collared cotton knit golf shirt.[2] Another sportswear company, Wright & Ditson, was founded in 1871 in Boston by George Wright and Henry A. Ditson, who had both owned sporting goods companies prior to their merger. Wright played baseball for the Boston Red Stockings National League team along with Alfred

G. Spalding, who also, with his brother, had founded a sporting goods company, in Chicago in the 1870s. The Spalding brothers' enterprise thrived, eventually buying out Wright & Ditson in 1891. The name continued into the 1940s, however, providing apparel and sporting goods to schools such as Mount Holyoke College and many others during the development of the gym suit.

Another early company, still in operation at the beginning of the twenty-first century, is Jantzen, founded in Portland, Oregon, in 1910. Begun as the Portland Knitting Company to produce heavy wool sweaters, socks, and gloves, it turned to the product it is still known for, bathing suits, after the Portland Rowing Club approached the owners to request a new kind of swimsuit that would keep the rowers warm in their early morning workouts on the water. The result, in 1913, was a striped one-piece wool ribbed knit suit, warm and stretchy, adapted from the hand-operated knitting machine for making ribbed cuffs, which the company was already using. Carl C. Jantzen, one of the original founders of the company in 1910, designed the suit, following, it would seem, the styles seen at the 1912 Olympics. The suit, which was the same for men and women, weighed eight pounds when wet. It was patented in 1921, the same year the red diving girl, first used as a catalogue logo, was adopted as the company's official trademark.[3]

These companies, all appearing in the years around the turn of the twentieth century, answered the needs of a sport-oriented public. All began small but by the 1920s were mass-producing their garments. It was mass production as much as anything else that led to an overall simplification in dress. Without the labor-intensive hand-cutting and sophisticated fitting of women's clothing that characterized fashion into the second decade of the twentieth century, manufacturers were freed from the expensive details that had defined their products. This move away from intricate draping and fitting and towards mass production allowed the manufacturers to make women's clothing that was simple, straight-cut, and loose on the body. Mass manufacturing, then, allowed cheaper, less contrived clothing for the masses, ushering in a whole new concept in dress. The companies that began to manufacture sports apparel during these years represented the wave of the future in American society, linking designers, manufacturers, and the retailers who happily sold the mass-produced goods to the public, and in doing so helped to create the rampant consumer culture of today.

In the years immediately prior to World War I, other forces that affected clothing were coming to the fore as well. America was not the only part of the world smitten by sports and their accompanying new look. Europe, too, was enthralled. In France, new and untried designers were playing with ideas borrowed from sport. Of them all, Coco Chanel would have the greatest long-term impact (though she was not, perhaps, the most popular in the early days of her career). Chanel created not only her own style of clothes but her own history as well. She was the mistress of an English nobleman, Boy Cappel, who, true to his upbringing and status, was a sportsman. During the years of their liaison, Chanel borrowed his sweaters and knit shirts and created new clothes for herself based on their simple lines. These knits, based strictly on sport apparel, called *tricots* in French, became the staple of her line, which blossomed after World War I. They were trim and unadorned, comfortable and easy, simple in style but expensive and elite. Other French designers responded to the sporting image as well, most notably Jean Patou, who created the innovative tennis dress first worn by Suzanne Lenglen in 1919. Patou got more coverage in the fashion magazines than Chanel did, but he had the misfortune to die young, whereas Chanel lived into energetic old age, reinventing herself once again in the 1950s.[4]

All the ingredients were in place: sports, new clothing from several different sources, and the publicity provided by the print media. But one last factor, more than any other, sold the ideas gleaned from sports to the public. That factor was the movies. Interestingly, the movies and women's competitive sports debuted on the scene within a few years of each other. The earliest movie appeared in 1896, three years after the introduction of basketball for women. By 1903 the first successful sustained movie, *The Great Train Robbery*, had grabbed the imagination of America, simultaneously giving birth to the Hollywood western and a moviegoing public whose avidity grew as the years went by. The invented world of the movies rapidly began to transform the tastes and attitudes of audiences everywhere.[5]

Around 1910 the fledgling movie industry relocated from New York and New Jersey to California to take advantage of a climate that allowed virtually nonstop production. By 1915 filmmakers were making movies of all kinds, and had helped to establish the center of the American film industry on the West Coast. Young directors chose young, beautiful women to tell their stories, creating as an unexpected by-product the cult of the movie star. This became obvious as early as the 1910s, when audiences started demanding to know the names of their favorite players, who had previously gone admired but unidentified. By the 1920s, all the world had embraced the productions and the stars, the young and the beautiful who wore wonderful clothes and moved in elegant surroundings. They even read about their favorite stars in the myriad movie magazines that mushroomed to accompany the film industry.[6] Many showed illustrations of the popular actors of the day in their own clothes or their own settings. The clothes, of course, were those worn in warm and sunny Los Angeles. They were often the casual clothing of the leisured well-to-do. But the movie magazine–buying public saw the stars as icons to be adored and copied, so the casual clothing of California and its movie colony became the dress of choice.

A good example of how Hollywood helped modernize clothing can be seen in the movies of Mack Sennett, who founded his film company, Keystone, in 1912. Keystone, best known today for its slapstick comedy embodied by the Keystone Kops, also delighted its audience with its youthful "Bathing Beauties," who figured prominently in Keystone films. At first they wore the "heavy skirty kind" of bathing dress, complete with bloomers, stockings and skirt, but soon the more daring appeared in modifications of the body-fitting men's swimsuits that had first been seen in the 1912 Olympics.[7] Jantzen was introducing its new one-piece knit suits in these same years. It seems clear that the movies helped delighted audiences accept the newer, barer, and more daring bathing suits long before they were more generally seen on the beaches of America.

Other clothing the "Beauties" wore, usually of their own choice at this time and ranging from homemade to designer-crafted, was equally influential. Audiences were already tuning in to the "looks" of their favorites. The movie magazines followed up with articles on the stars, their lives, and their clothing choices. By the late 1920s, young, slim, and beautiful actresses such as Clara Bow in *It* (1927) and Joan Crawford in *Our Dancing Daughters* (1928) insisted on costumes that would show off their slender, trim bodies. The clothes they chose to showcase their youthful perfection were slim-fitted patterned sweaters, pert pleated skirts, now short enough to barely cover the knee, even men's dress shirts and jodhpurs, tailored blazers and skirts— clothes for sport. Suddenly, following their lead, the baggy, waistless dresses of the 1920s gave way to the svelte, fitted outfits of the 1930s. And the category of sportswear was born. Even the gym suit was transformed from the bulky middy and bloomers into an attractive tennis-dress style in imitation of the fashionable tennis dresses that were so popular on the courts at the time.

In addition, trousers for women finally found a place in the world of public clothing. Although it would take another half century, into the 1980s, before pants-wearing women were accepted anywhere, everywhere, without censure, knickerbockers and beach pajamas, which had developed from the bloomers of the previous decades, opened the door in the 1920s.[8] They were never worn in public and even into the 1930s, only in private or non-urban leisure settings. Wearing tailored trousers in public was the daring choice of the unconventional few: Marlene Dietrich wore them to shock, to blur the boundaries of sexuality and gender. Katharine Hepburn wore them as an unquestioned expression of her upper-class, sport-oriented upbringing. She was criticized for it.[9] By the end of the 1930s, though, Hepburn occasionally wore trousers in her movies, and looked completely at ease—and acceptable—in them. Her unconventional and unconcerned approach to style had helped to convince the public that trousers on women were not unthinkable after all—predating the defense-worker pants of World War II by several years.

Thus, the merging of public and private was finally complete. It had taken almost a century for this to happen. The comfortable, practical, fashionable clothing that emerged in the 1930s is now regarded as American Style. Its antecedents were many. But once it appeared—with its individual items based on men's clothing, and the clothing for sports—shirts, sweaters, jackets, and skirts, and finally trousers as well—it never went away. In a fashion world that revolves around frenetic change, one that promotes new fads and fashions every year, even every season, this stability is almost unbelievable. Yet the easy and elegant look of a young Katharine Hepburn in her trousers, boat shoes, and tailored shirts, waiting on set for her call, is the look of today. Now the entire world wears American sportswear. It is the final legacy of those intrepid young women in the early nineteenth century who came outdoors to play.

$$\boxed{\text{NOTES}}$$

PART ONE INTRODUCTION

1. Mount Holyoke, opened in 1837, is the oldest institution of higher education for women still in existence. It became a degree-granting college in the 1880s.

2. Stephen Hardy, *How Boston Played: Sport, Recreation, and Community, 1865–1915* (Boston: Northeastern University Press, 1982), 62.

3. Steve Brouwer, *Sharing the Pie: A Citizen's Guide to Wealth and Power* (New York: Henry Holt & Co., 1998), excerpted in http://www.thirdworldtraveler.com/Economics.SharingPie.html (accessed February 5, 2002).

4. Ibid., 144.

5. Mary Queen of Scots in the mid-sixteenth century was known to have been a golfer, taking the game with her when she became queen of France.

6. Website of the Nova Scotia Golf Association. www.nsga.ns.ca/NSGA_Hist_Canada.htm (accessed February 5, 2002).

7. Ibid.

8. For information on clothing for equestrian sports, see Alexander Mackay-Smith et al., *Man and the Horse* (New York: Metropolitan Museum of Art and Simon and Schuster, 1984); and, for summaries of both equestrian costume and golf wear, *The Encyclopedia of Clothing and Fashion* (New York: Charles Scribner and Sons, 2005).

1. FACTORS OF CHANGE

1. The Beechers were a remarkable family, comparable to the eighteenth-century Adams and twentieth-century Kennedy families. The patriarch, Lyman, one of the core of Congregational preachers in New England notable for their pivotal roles in the Second Great Awakening, was born in New Haven in 1775. As the author of *Uncle Tom's Cabin* (1851), Harriet is undoubtedly the best known. But Lyman fathered twelve other children, several of whom became stars in their own right. Catharine, the

eldest, founded successful schools for girls in both Hartford and Cincinnati, and wrote *A Treatise on Domestic Economy*, published in 1841, a best-selling domestic guide throughout the remainder of the nineteenth century. Many of the siblings were authors and educators; one would become the grandmother of the humanist and early feminist Charlotte Perkins Gilman, author of "The Yellow Wallpaper." Henry Ward Beecher, one of the youngest children of Lyman's first wife, was the preacher of his generation, a nineteenth-century equivalent to Billy Graham. By 1847, while still in his thirties, he was the pastor of a 2,500-member congregation in Brooklyn. His sermons were so popular they were published weekly. Beecher Family Papers, 1822–1903, MS 0509, Mount Holyoke College Archives and Special Collections, South Hadley, Mass.

2. Foster Rhea Dulles, *America Learns to Play* (New York: D. Appleton-Century Co., 1940), 87–91.

3. Quoted ibid., 85.

4. Ibid.

5. John F. Kasson, *Amusing the Millions* (New York: Hill & Wang, 1978), 4.

6. Ibid., 13–15; *Encyclopedia Britannica*, s.v. "Frederick Law Olmsted"; Olmsted and Vaux remained partners for close to twenty years, sharing the work on many of the park designs. See www.fredericklawolmsted.com (accessed February 22, 2002).

7. Klasson, *Amusing*, 15.

8. U.S. Census data, 1871.

9. See Ann Douglas Wood, "'The Fashionable Diseases': Women's Complaints and Their Treatment in Nineteenth-Century America," in Mary Hartman and Lois Banner, eds, *Clio's Consciousness Raised* (New York: Harper & Row, 1974), 1–22.

10. All information on Elizabeth Blackwell is from an on-line version of an exhibition on Blackwell held at the National Library of Medicine, National Institutes of Health, Bethesda, Md., January 23–September 4, 1999. www.nlm.nih.gov/hmd/blackwell

11. Regina Morantz, "The Lady and Her Physician," in Hartman and Banner, *Clio's Consciousness Raised*, 46.

12. Ibid., 48–49. See also Steven J. Peitzman, *A New and Untried Course: Woman's Medical College and Medical College of Pennsylvania, 1850–1998* (Piscataway, N.J.: Rutgers University Press, 2000).

13. *Godey's* (January 1866): 91.

14. On Blackwell, see National Medical Library website. Her book, *The Laws of Life, with Special Reference to the Physical Education of Girls,* was published in 1852 (New York: George P. Putnam). *Peterson's Magazine* (November 1852) featured a four-page article written by Charles J. Peterson himself on "Mrs. Blackwell's" work (232–35).

15. *Peterson's Magazine* (November 1852): 234.

16. Ibid., 233.

17. See www.princeton.edu/~mcbrown/display/cole.html.

18. See www4.umdnj.edu/camlbweb/sjmedhist/sjwomen.html.

19. These included Abba Goold Woolson, a champion of dress reform whom we will meet in Part Two.

20. *Godey's* (January 1864): 93–95.

21. Ibid. (July 1864): 85.

22. Morantz, "The Lady and Her Physician," 42, 52.

23. *Godey's* (November 1860): 462. See Hartman and Banner, *Clio's Consciousness Raised,* for essays by Ann Douglas Wood, Carroll Smith-Rosenburg, Regina Morantz, and Linda Gordon for insight into the Victorian woman, her gynecological problems and their treatment.

24. See, for example, Nancy Woloch, "Sarah Hale and The Lady's Magazine" and "Promoting Woman's Sphere, 1800–1860," in *Women and the American Experience* (New York: Arno Press, 1974), 97–150. For a history of women's magazines in America, see also Mary Ellen Zuckerman, *A History of Popular Women's Magazines in the United States, 1792–1995* (Westport, Con.: Greenwood Press, 1998), and Zuckerman's compilation, *Sources on the History of Women's Magazines, 1792–1960: An Annotated Bibliography* (New York: Greenwood Press, 1991); Frank Luther Mott, *A History of American Magazines* (Cambridge, Mass.: Belknap Press of Harvard University Press, ca. 1957–ca. 1968); Ellen Gruber Garvey, *The Adman in the Parlor: Magazines and the Gendering of Consumer Culture, 1880s to 1910s* (New York: Oxford University Press, 1996); Helen Damon-Moore, *Magazines for the Millions: Gender and Commerce in the Ladies' Home Journal and the Saturday Evening Post, 1880–1910* (Albany: State University of New York Press, ca. 1994).

25. *Harper's Weekly*: September 4, 1858, 568, "The Bathe at Newport"; January 28, 1860, 56–57, "Skating on the Ladies' Skating Pond in Central Park, New York." In all, Homer created 147 original woodcuts for *Harper's*.

26. In 2001 dollars, this would amount to approximately $5,500. Here and throughout, all comparative dollar amounts are calculated courtesy of www.westegg.com/inflation.

27. All information on Howe, Singer, and the sewing machine may be found in Phyllis Tortora and Keith Eubank, *The Survey of Historic Costume,* 3d ed. (New York: Fairchild, 1998), 302; Scientific American On-Line, www.history.rochester.edu/Scientific_American/mystery/howe.htm; the National Museum of American History, www.si.org; and the website of the International Sewing Machine Collectors' Society, www.geocities.com/RodeoDrive/6561/Singer/the_singer_history.htm.

28. *Godey's* (February 1863): 194.

29. Ibid. (March 1863): 201.

30. Claudia B. Kidwell and Margaret C. Christman, *Suiting Everyone: The Democratization of Clothing in America* (Washington, D.C.: Smithsonian Institution Press, 1974), 75–77.

31. Susan Porter Benson, *Counter Cultures: Saleswomen, Managers, and Customers in the American Department Store, 1890–1940* (Urbana: University of Illinois Press, 1986), chap. 1, "A New Kind of Store." It must be remembered that at that time Macy's was a single store. In 2001 terms, $1 million equals almost $13 million. Richard H. Edwards, *Tales of the Observer* (Boston: Jordan Marsh Co., ca. 1950); Kidwell and Christman, *Suiting Everyone.*

32. Kidwell and Christman, *Suiting Everyone,* 137.

33. This new knit cloth, introduced in the late 1870s, was named for Lily Langtry, social climber, actress, and mistress of the Prince of Wales, who was known as "The Jersey Lily." Perhaps the most celebrated of the Beautiful People of her day, she came from the Isle of Jersey. See Phyllis Cunnington and Alan Mansfield, *English Costume for Sports and Outdoor Recreation: From the Sixteenth to the Nineteenth Centuries* (New York: Barnes & Noble, 1970), 89.

2. WOMEN MOVE OUT-OF-DOORS

1. For two early proponents of "trickle-down theory," see Thorstein Veblen, *Theory of the Leisure Class* (1899; reprint, New York: Random House, 1961); and Georg Simmel, "Fashion," *International Quarterly* 10 (1904): 130–55.

2. Foster Rhea Dulles, *America Learns to Play* (New York: D. Appleton-Century Co., 1940), 164, quoting diarist Samuel Dexter Ward.

3. They still exist, now as German culture clubs, as much as anything else, for example, in Springfield, Massachusetts.

4. Fred Eugene Leonard, *History of Physical Education* (Philadelphia: Lea & Febiger, 1923), 225.

5. See Mr. Baseball website, www.mrbaseball.com/history; www.mrbaseball .com/hoboken2, for a complete history of the game. From the time of its formation in September 1845, the Knickerbocker Base Ball Club regarded Elysian Fields as its home field and played there every Monday and Thursday afternoon for the term of the club's forty-year existence. Clearly, these young men were of the leisured class rather than the working class, at least in the beginning. So dominant was the Knickerbocker Club through the 1850s that it helped to organize many of the early baseball clubs and transformed Elysian Fields into the first great center of baseball activity in the United States. By 1859, eight teams participated in the National Association of Base Ball Players (the first baseball organization in the United States and a forerunner of the National League) and played regularly each week at Elysian Fields. Dulles, *America Learns to Play*, also gives a clear background of the rise in sports.

6. Dulles, *America Learns to Play*, 187.

7. David Park Curry, "Winslow Homer and Croquet," *Antiques Magazine* (July 1984): 154, quoting from the 1865 guide "How to Play Croquet."

8. Unless otherwise indicated, all references to the history of croquet, including quotations, may be found in David Park Curry, *Winslow Homer: The Croquet Game* (New Haven: Yale University Art Gallery, 1984), unpaginated. Curry tells us that *paille maille*, eventually anglicized into Pall Mall, gave its name to the London street that had started life as a playing ground for the game.

9. For the history of the lawn mower, see the website of the British Old Lawn-mower Club, http://www.artizan.demon.co.uk/olc/mowhist.htm. My thanks to James B. Ricci of the Reel Lawn Mower History and Preservation Project @ North Farms, Haydenville, Massachusetts, for his additional history and for verifying the link between the lawn mower and tennis. He states: "The entry of the horse, wearing oversize leather booties to prevent lawn damage, drawing a very wide reel mower allowed vast estate lawns and playing fields to be more quickly and cheaply cut. The sheep were even displaced from the job of keeping the golf course fairway short."

10. *Peterson's Magazine* (July 1870): 76.

11. An elevator was a device consisting of series of rings sewn into the underside of a skirt or petticoat through which strings were threaded, then pulled and tied in place to hike up the skirt in evenly spaced and artful flounces.

12. Mayne Reid, *Croquet: A Treatise with notes and commentaries* (New York, 1869), quoted in Curry, *Winslow Homer.*

13. "Croquet," *Harper's Bazar*, October 24, 1868, 827. The magazine's name was spelled with a single "a" until 1901, when it became *Harper's Bazaar*, by which it is still known.

14. One of the consistencies of the fashion plates of the time is the appearance of the tiny female foot. Even though the shoes of the period (still referred to at that time as "straights" because they did not distinguish between right and left) look small to the twenty-first-century eye, it must be remembered that the sole was narrow, but the soft leather or cloth of the uppers "gave" with the weight of the foot and expanded over the edges of the sole.

15. *Godey's* (January 1867): 107.

16. A. F. M. Willich, *The Domestic Encyclopedia, or a Dictionary of Facts and Useful Knowledge* (Philadelphia: Abraham Small, 1821).

17. Colin McDowell, *Shoes* (New York: Rizzoli, 1989), 143; June Swann, *Shoes* (London: M. T. Batsford, 1982), 41–42.

18. *Bloomingdale's Illustrated 1886 Catalogue* (New York: Dover Publications, 1988), 75. Webster applied for a patent to attach rubber soles to shoes in 1832. Rubber galoshes had also been developed in the United States before 1836 and came into wider use in the 1840s. The lightweight rubbers that Bloomingdale's advertised were widespread in the 1880s. Called "softs," they were used in Britain in the country during summertime, and before this time as bathing shoes, known "by the ugly name of plimsolls." Swann, *Shoes*, 40–56.

19. Dulles, *America Learns to Play*, 192.

20. See *Godey's* (December 1863): 566–68, for all quotations.

21. Ibid. (February 1864): 200–201.

22. Ibid. (March 1864): 280.

23. Ibid. (May 1864): 495.

24. Ibid. (January 1868): 100.

25. François Boucher, *Histoire du costume* (Paris: Flammarion, 1983), 376.

26. Ibid., 380.

27. Alison Gernsheim, *Fashion and Reality* (London: Faber and Faber, 1963), 45.

28. Boucher, *Histoire du costume*, 380.

29. *Godey's* (May 1864): 495.

30. Millia Davenport, *The Book of Costume* (New York: Crown Publishers, 1976), 902–3. The actual year of the appearance of Mme. Demorest's *Mirror of Fashion* is in some doubt. Joy Spanabel Emery, in her history of paper patterns, "Dreams on Paper," in Barbara Burman, ed., *The Culture of Sewing* (Oxford: Berg, 1999), suggests the date was 1860 (238).

31. *Godey's* (May 1864): 495.

32. Ibid. (February 1864): 211.

33. All quotations ibid. A Garibaldi was a loose, baggy, tucked-in shirt, usually of red wool, copied from the ones worn by the Italian hero Giuseppe Garibaldi in his battle for unity and reform in Italy. Early in his colorful career, Garibaldi had formed an Italian legion in South America, the original "Redshirts." The undisputed superhero of his day, he spent time in South America, the United States (in exile), and several parts of Europe, always fighting against tyranny. His greatest exploit was to lead an expedition of a thousand men (*i mille*) to assist a revolt in Sicily in 1860. Their uniform, such as it was, was the red shirt. The revolt fizzled, but Garibaldi himself was remarkably successful, and was proclaimed dictator of Sicily in the name of King Victor Emmanuel II, a positon he refused to accept. A prototype of later dictators, his lack of intellect was compensated for by his extraordinary dash and charisma. No wonder his red shirts became the fashion of choice in the 1860s. The Garibaldi was usually worn with a long skirt. The one mentioned in *Godey's* would have been shortened to the knee because it was to be worn with Turkish pants, which were long, baggy trousers gathered at the ankle.

34. Although I say this purely anecdotally, so many women have reported this to me over the years that I have no doubt of its veracity.

35. *Godey's* (March 1867): 295.

3. TAKING UP TENNIS

1. This history of tennis is taken from the following essays in Allison Danzig and Peter Schwed, eds., *The Fireside Book of Tennis* (New York: Simon and Schuster, 1972): "Major Walter C. Wingfield, Inventor of the Game," by Parke Cummings (9–14); "Sphairistike, History of the United States Lawn Tennis Association," by Allison Danzig (14–20); and "The Gentler Sex," by Edward C. Potter Jr. (75–78); also Richard Schickel, *The World of Tennis* (New York: Random House, 1975), 32–37.

2. Cummings, "Major Wingfield," 11.

3. Ibid., 13.

4. Henry Hall, ed., *The Tribune Book of Open-Air Sports, prepared by The New York Tribune with the aid of Acknowledged Experts* (New York: Tribune Association, 1887), 105–6.

5. Foster Rhea Dulles, *America Learns to Play* (New York: D. Appleton-Century Co., 1940), 192.

6. My thanks to James B. Ricci of the Reel Lawn Mower History and Preservation Project @ North Farms, Haydenville, Massachusetts, for information on lawn mowers and the sign at Wimbledon. My first clue to the importance of this homely machine came from Peter Ustinov's commentary on NBC during the 1986 Wimbledon finals (July 6, 1986) as he described the history of tennis. Time and again we are reminded that technology enabled the mass production of machinery and equipment that underlay the pastimes of leisure.

7. Schickel, *World of Tennis*, 32.

8. Website of the Lawn Tennis Association of Great Britain, www.lta.org.uk/projects/histen.htm (accessed February, 6, 2002). One correction: Goodyear invented the vulcanization process in 1839, not the 1850s as suggested by the website.

9. Phillis Cunnington and Alan Mansfield, *English Costume for Sports and Outdoor Recreation: From the Sixteenth to the Nineteenth Centuries* (New York: Barnes & Noble, 1970), 89.

10. An equivalent price for the outfit with the silk blouse in 2001 dollars is $331.20—no small amount. Even the cheviot (cotton twill) version at $13.75 would cost $260.23 in 2001 dollars, a surprising difference of some $70 in equivalent terms between the two blouses.

11. Claudia B. Kidwell and Margaret C. Christman, *Suiting Everyone: The Democratization of Clothing in America* (Washington, D.C.: Smithsonian Institution Press, 1974), 142.

12. Potter, "Gentler Sex," 75.

13. "Aesthetic" dress was so called because it was designed by the artists connected with the Aesthetic movement in England and worn by their wives and mistresses, who often modeled for them. It fits into the general category of fashion history known as "reform dress." It was an attempt to recall the simplicity of preindustrial Europe, and to reject the fashionable constraint in women's clothes in the second half of the nineteenth century—hoops, bustles, corsets, tight fit, and all—in favor of a sort of flowing medieval pastiche. It came into its own in the 1880s after being gently ridiculed by Gilbert and Sullivan in *Patience*, first performed in 1881.

14. *The Delineator* (August 1891): 78.

15. Colin McDowell, *Shoes* (New York: Rizzoli, 1989), 143.

16. *The Delineator* (July 1892): 68.

17. Anne Buck, "Foundations of the Active Woman," *La Belle Epoque*, proceedings of the Costume Society Spring Conference, 1967, 63.

18. Potter, "Gentler Sex," 75.

19. Jeane Hoffman, "The Sutton Sisters," in Danzig and Schwed, *Fireside Book of Tennis*, 74.

20. Potter, "Gentler Sex," 77.

21. Robert H. Lauer and Jeannette C. Lauer, *Fashion Power* (Englewood Cliffs, N.J.: Prentice-Hall, 1981), 89.

22. *Minneapolis Star and Tribune*, June 28, 1985.

23. The armsceye is the opening in the bodice for the inset of the sleeve. In the 1880s it had achieved the highest position it ever would and still allow for some movement of the arm, and was refined into a perfect circle. This particular cut permitted movement but put fierce strain on the upper sleeve as well as the front and back bodice where the sleeves were attached.

24. Blazers were so called because of their stripes, or blazes. They usually indicated the colors of the wearer's club.

25. "The Women's Colleges of the United States. No. 4. A Girl's Life and Work at Bryn Mawr," *The Delineator* (August 1894): 213.

26. *The Delineator* (August 1894): xxviii. This ad for a tennis manual offered every kind of advice needed to play the game: a history of the game, rules, development of play, descriptions of the court, implements, serviceable dress, even a chapter on tournaments and how to conduct them.

27. Elizabeth Ewing, *History of Twentieth-Century Fashion* (London: B. T. Batsford, 1974), 76–77.

28. Quoted in James Laver, *Modesty in Dress* (Boston: Houghton Mifflin, 1969), 144–45.

4. BATHING AND SWIMMING

1. James Laver, *Modesty in Dress* (Boston: Houghton Mifflin, 1969), 140.

2. See Claudia B. Kidwell, *Women's Bathing and Swimming Costume in the United States* (Washington, D.C.: U.S. Government Printing Office, 1963), for a full history of swimwear; and Barbara A. Schreier, "Sporting Wear," in Claudia Brush Kidwell and Valerie Steele, eds., *Men and Women Dressing the Part* (Washington, D.C.: Smithsonian Institution Press, 1989), 117.

3. See Cindy S. Aron, *Working at Play* (New York: Oxford University Press, 1999), for a history of leisure, resorts, and vacation spots into the twentieth century. Her chapter 3, "'Through the streets in bathing costumes': Resort Vacations, 1850–1900," describes much seaside resort behavior and clothing in the latter half of the nineteenth century.

4. Jennie Holliman, *American Sports (1785–1835)* (Durham, N.C.: Seeman Press, 1931), 168.

5. Kidwell, *Women's Bathing and Swimming Costume*, 8–9.

6. *Godey's* (September 1873): 292.

7. Paula D. Welch, *History of American Physical Education and Sport* (Springfield, Ill.: Charles C. Thomas, 1981), 226, 231.

8. "Bathing suit" as a term appeared first in the 1880s, when any matching skirt and bodice combination was referred to as a suit even though it was designed as a two-piece dress. Throughout the next few decades, "bathing costume" and "bathing dress" were interchangeable terms.

9. My own grandparents, both born in the 1880s, always referred to any swimming activity as "going in for a dip." I had always thought it a quaint phrase until I realized while doing this research that their term quite literally described their activity. "Swimming" to them did, in fact, amount to dipping and little more.

10. *Frank Leslie's Ladies Gazette of Fashion* (June 1854): 103.

11. Quoted in Kidwell, *Women's Bathing and Swimming Costume*, 17.

12. *Godey's* (July 1864): 96. Moreen was a sturdy ribbed fabric of either wool or cotton, often with an embossed finish—a cross between moiré and velveteen. That it was used for both clothing and upholstery indicates just how sturdy it was.

13. Ibid.

14. *Harper's Bazar*, July 10, 1869.

15. A good example of this practice may be seen in *The Young Girl's Book*, published in New York sometime in the earlier decades of the nineteenth century (no date is given). The illustrations, to judge by the clothes, all date from the 1820s and 1830s. A series of calisthenics and another of dance steps are illustrated with the (same) figure wearing a simple higher-waisted, relatively short bell-skirted dress with huge, full balloon sleeves to the elbow—typical of the early 1830s. This same set of illustrations

is used again in a series of articles on exercises for health and beauty in *Godey's Lady's Book* (1848). My thanks to Susan Greene for *The Young Girls' Book*.

16. This bathing suit is yet another example of copying. The illustration appeared first in *Godey's* in July 1870, then again the next month in *Peterson's*. Needless to say, no acknowledgment was given. One can only wonder where it had started out.

17. *Peterson's Magazine* (August 1870): 159.

18. *Godey's* (July 1871): 43.

19. All the references to flannel, which was made from either cotton or wool, almost definitely refer to the wool version. The clue is provided by the alternate choices, often serge, as here. This was the era when wool next to the skin was preferable for warmth, especially when it was wet—never mind that it would be very heavy for the purpose.

20. *Harper's Bazar*, June 13, 1896, 503.

21. Mary R. Melendy, M.D., Ph.D., *The Perfect Woman* (Bay City, Mich.: H. H. Taylor Publishing Co., 1901), 319.

22. *The Delineator*, July 1890, 65.

23. Kidwell, *Women's Bathing and Swimming Costume*, 24.

24. Indeed, even though the imprint is Bay City, Michigan, that means very little at this time. The whole book may well have been English. I have found entire books in special collections copied, at a later date, with the title changed as well as the publisher and place of publication but in all else exactly the same. The concept of plagiarism as a sin, or at least as a crime, did not yet exist.

25. *Harper's Bazar*, July 3, 1897, 543.

26. Kidwell, *Women's Bathing and Swimming Costume*, 25.

27. See photographs in *Torontonensis* (the yearbook of the University of Toronto), 1900, for a comparison between Kellerman's swimsuit and the male gymnasts' outfits.

28. *Ladies' Home Journal* (August 1910): 11. Kellerman provides a glimpse of how far the ideal image of women has shifted in the ensuing century. She justified her figure-revealing suit by declaring that Dr. Dudley Sargent of health and fitness measurement fame had taken her measurements and pronounced them to be "nearer the correct proportions than he had ever seen." She was five feet and three and three-quarters inches tall, and weighed 137 pounds, with body measurements of 35.2", 26.2", 37.8".

29. Quoted in Kidwell, *Women's Bathing and Swimming Costume*, 26.

30. Personal interview, Evelyn W. Campbell, July 19, 1985, speaking of early years at Cawaja Beach on Georgian Bay in Ontario. "Mercerized" refers to a process developed in the mid-nineteenth century for preshrinking cotton thread. It gave an added luster to the fabric. Sateen is also a cotton, woven to give an even greater sheen, much like satin.

31. I own two suits from this period, one wool and the other cotton. Although the cotton feels better against the skin, the wool suit provides much more stretch and give. The cotton suit just seems heavy and inert. As with an old T-shirt once the cotton has reached its final shape after many washings, nothing in the world can change it.

32. Personal interview, August 3, 1985.

33. Joan Ryan, unknown source, late 1970s. The suit was expensive indeed: $28 would equal about $350 today.

34. Ibid.

35. Kidwell, *Women's Bathing and Swimming Costume*, 47.

36. Ryan interview.

37. Ibid.

28. In the spring of 1999, movie star Julia Roberts shocked the world when she was photographed with underarm hair in clear view as she waved to her fans at a London premiere. It created a sensation; she removed the hair. Dozens of websites and chat pages (some sixty-nine in 2002) around the world worried over the question, should she or shouldn't she?

5. WOMEN ENTER THE OLYMPICS

1. One remembers the flak tennis player Anne White received for wearing her white body suit at Wimbledon in 1985—not so long ago.

2. *Time*, the *New York Times Magazine*, and many others made these claims. The special issue of the *Times*, "Women Muscle In" (June 23, 1996), by its very title denotes the ambivalence that still exists. The phrase "muscle in" suggests that women were unwelcome outsiders, even bullies, although the articles were very supportive of women's Olympic status. It is not just the Olympics that have given women opportunities: soccer and basketball have, too. *Newsweek* did a better job in its cover headline of July 19, 1999, with its empowering photo of Brandi Chastain pumping her fists after her U.S. soccer team's final victory: "Girls Rule!" (Of course, many women would take exception to the word "girls," regarding it as demeaning for grown women.)

3. David Wallechinski, *Book of the Olympics* (New York: Penguin Books, 1984), x.

4. Most books and articles brush over the rarity of women in the Olympics up to about 1924. *Grace and Glory: A Century of Women in the Olympics* (Chicago: Triumph Books, 1996) is an exception. Even here, though, the only mention of clothing is in the caption for a photograph of Annette Kellerman in her "'indecent' one-piece bathing suit."

5. Adrienne Blue, *Faster, Higher, Further: Women's Triumphs and Disasters at the Olympics* (London: Virago Press, 1988), 1. It is interesting to note that at least one biography of Coubertin never mentions women or his thoughts about them at all. See John J. MacAloon, *This Great Symbol* (Chicago: University of Chicago Press, 1981).

6. Ellen W. Gerber et al., *The American Woman in Sport* (Reading, Mass.: Addison-Wesley, 1974), 137–38; Uriel Simri, "The Development of Female Participation in the Modern Olympic Games," *Stadion* 6 (1980): 188.

7. Mary Henson Leigh, "The Evolution of Women's Participation in the Summer Olympic Games, 1900–1948" (Ph.D. diss., Ohio State University, 1974), 56.

8. Coubertin, "L'Éducation des jeunes enfants et des jeunes filles" (1902), quoted ibid., 56, 58.

9. Ibid., 77. Here Leigh quotes from a novel based on Coubertin, but the sentiments were very much his own, as all accounts attest (see particularly Simri, "Development," 188–89). Coubertin was in the overwhelming majority in believing that sports were

detrimental to women's femininity, as an article by the American physician Arabella Kenealy, titled "Woman as Athlete," detailed in 1899. With the weight of her medical training behind her, she stated that if women spent themselves in sports, they would have nothing left over to fulfill their "womanly duties." Even a woman's appearance was changed by sport, she reported, and not necessarily for the better: her glance became too unwavering and direct, "the haze, the elusiveness, the subtle suggestion of the face [or, to Coubertin, the mystery] are gone." Stephanie L. Twin, *Out of the Bleachers* (Old Westbury, N.Y.: Feminist Press, 1979), 44.

10. All the statistics on numbers of participants in this chapter are taken from Blue, *Faster, Higher*, ix, unless otherwise noted.

11. Leigh, "Evolution," 107, cites an article by Casper Whitney that appeared in the April 1900 issue of *Outing* which even then conjectured on the reasons for the confusion and poor management of the Paris Games. Histories of the Olympics are at odds about this second Olympiad, even as to the numbers of women who participated. Some, like Joanna Davenport, "The Women's Movement into the Olympic Games, 1900–1926," *Journal of Physical Education and Recreation* 49, no. 3 (1978): 58–60, and Gerber et al., *American Woman in Sport*, suggest that only six participated. Another, Wallechinski, *Book of the Olympics*, states that there were eleven. Reet Howell, *Her Story in Sport* (West Point, N.Y.: Leisure Press, 1982), 212, citing Simri, "Development," puts the number at twelve. All agree that, in Howell's words, it was a "lackadaisical" affair.

12. Wallechinski, *Book of the Olympics*, xvii; William Oscar Johnson, "100 Years of Glory" (Centennial Olympic Games Official Souvenir Program, 1996), 62; Paula D. Welch and Harold A. Lerch, *History of American Physical Education and Sport* (Springfield, Ill.: Charles C. Thomas, 1981), 289–90; MacAloon, *Great Symbol*, 274; *The Olympic Story* (Danbury, Conn.: Grolier Enterprises, 1979), 41.

13. Paula Welch and Margaret D. Costa, "A Century of Olympic Competition," in Margaret D. Costa and Sharon R. Guthrie, eds., *Women and Sport* (Champaign, Ill.: Human Kinetics, 1994), 136.

14. Johnson, "100 Years," 62–63. Abbott later married, settled in New York City, and became friends with Charles Dana Gibson, who drew her portrait in 1903; she thus became the Gold Medal Gibson Girl.

15. Welch and Costa, "Century," 124.

16. Leigh, "Evolution," 58. In spite of his enthusiasm, the letter writer still firmly upheld Coubertin's views of women in sports. "I approve of what the Baron de Coubertin. . . has written on this subject [of equality of the sexes]," he declared.

17. Archery had been a ladylike pastime for at least a century, as images throughout the nineteenth century attest. Part of its appeal was the elegant arrangement of graceful clothing, straight silhouetted body, and feminine beauty highlighted by a woman's skill (or lack thereof) in pulling the bowstring. Even the movies, which so often get period details wrong, portrayed archery with accuracy and delight in the 1996 film version of *Emma*, as Gwyneth Paltrow in the title role shows off her deadly aim.

18. Welch and Lerch, *History*, 159.

19. Jennifer Hargreaves, "Women and the Olympic Phenomenon," in Alan Tomlinson and Garry Whannel, eds., *Five Ring Circus* (London: Pluto Press, 1984), 56–57.

20. Wallechinski, *Book of the Olympics*, 155, 550; Kathleen E. McCrone, *Playing the Game* (Lexington: University of Kentucky Press, 1988), 187; Hargreaves, "Women and the Olympic Phenomenon," 56–57.

21. Leigh, "Evolution," 111, quoting *London Daily Telegraph*, July 14, 1908. The outfits, according to an extant photograph, were very much like the American gymnastic suits of the time, though different in color. In Part Two I discuss gymnastic dress at length.

22. See Patricia Campbell Warner, "The Gym Slip: The Origins of the English Schoolgirl Tunic," *Dress* 22 (1995): 45–58, for a brief discussion.

23. One wonders how widely disseminated the photographs taken of this team were at the time. Since the outfits appeared in conjunction with the Olympics, it stands to reason that they were indeed much reported on and much seen. Other women were wearing knee-length skirts for sports activities as early as 1910 (see Part Two), so the idea of short skirts was "out there." Of course, they did not become accepted as fashion wear until the mid- to late 1920s, half a decade after the famous Patou tennis dress worn by Suzanne Lenglen at Wimbledon. Chanel admitted to being influenced by sports clothing, but only by men's, as early as the 1910s, though it would have been difficult for her to admit that she was influenced by other styles for women. Nevertheless, if women's early dress for sport provided new ideas for more mainstream fashion, it would have taken at least a decade for such a compelling change to be accepted across an entire population.

24. Harry Gordon, *Australia and the Olympic Games* (St. Lucia: University of Queensland Press, 1994), 75. The information in this chapter on the Australian women's struggle to enter the Olympic Games and the societal reaction to it comes from Gordon's fascinating book.

25. Few even noticed. This was Jim Thorpe's Olympics, and his superb performance, with its dark aftermath, overshadowed everything else.

26. The other fourteen were tennis players. Simri, "Development," 191–92.

27. The story of Fanny Durack and Mina Wiley, their travails and success, is told in Harry Gordon, "Here Come the Girls," in *Australia and the Olympic Games*, 75–89, quotation 80. A parallel American controversy over gymnastic dress was going on at the same time at Mount Holyoke College and other schools around the country (continuing in some places as late as the 1970s, where girls were admonished to cover up their gym suits with coats as they moved from one building to another).

28. This bikini-style bottom was known as "athletes' swimming drawers," or simply "athletes'." Richard Rutt claims that they were made primarily from cotton twill. They first appeared in the 1880s, but by the 1890s they were made from sateen (a kind of cotton), jersey (wool), cotton, flannelette, or even silk. Drawstrings tied the waist and the legs when needed. For an excellent history of men's swimming costume in England, see Richard Rutt, "The Englishman's Swimwear," *Costume*, no. 24 (1990): 69–84.

29. Claudia Kidwell, "Women's Bathing and Swimming Costume in the United States," Paper 64, Bulletin 250, Museum of History and Technology (1969), esp. 25–26. Kidwell mentions a woman's silk bathing suit of the 1920s, but it was designed more for fashion than competition.

30. This is an excellent example of how sports dress is first designed and introduced for speed in the Olympics, and later becomes mainstream fashion. We have seen this often in our own times, notably with bicycle shorts.

31. *New York Times*, July 19, 1913, quoted by Welch and Lerch, *History*, 292, who admit that "few women except for mavericks such as Ida Schnall dared to openly defy the powerful Sullivan." Few men, either, as we shall see.

32. *New York Times*, January 18, 1914, 1.

33. Welch and Lerch, *History*, 295–96.

34. Leigh, "Evolution," 128, 129, from minutes of AAU Annual Convention, 1914, as reported in *New York Times*, November 22, 1914.

35. Leigh, "Evolution," 131.

36. Ellen W. Gerber, *The American Woman in Sport* (Reading, Mass.: Addison-Wesley, 1974), 35.

37. Soule told *Time* that in 1920 she was "just an eighth-grader from Brooklyn Heights competing for the Women's Swimming Association of New York." *Time* 148, no. 1 special edition (Summer 1996): 96.

38. The men were labeled "sharks."

39. The *New York Times*, August 22, 1920, shows two European swimmers who had won races in Berlin and Paris that year, both wearing the utilitarian suits, as does a July 4, 1920, ad for a girls' summer camp showing a diver. A Stewart & Co. ad in the same July 4 edition, however, offers a dropped-waist, skirted "Black Surf Satin Bathing Suit in attractive belted model, with hanging pockets and armlets. The edges are trimmed with contrasting colored piping. Sizes 34 to 46. 4.75." Listed in the same ad, along with other price ranges for bathing suits, are tights, from $1.00 to $12.75. The illustration shows the model with stockings (or tights) rolled to the knee, and worn with cross-gartered bathing shoes. She sports a natty brimmed bathing hat.

40. Ibid., March 31, 1914, 9.

41. Welch and Costa, "Century," 126.

42. Accounts of the numbers in the early years vary. Generally, though, by 1920, some 9,300 men had participated in the Olympics since 1896, in comparison to 175 women. By anyone's account, women made up fewer than 2 percent of the whole during these first six Olympics.

43. The *New York Times*, August 30, 1920, 10.

44. Leigh, "Evolution," 306; Welch and Costa, "Century," 126.

45. Leigh, "Evolution," 306.

46. Ibid., 143.

47. Estimated figures from Jere Longman, "How the Women Won," in *New York Times Magazine*, special edition, "Women Muscle In," June 23, 1996, 24.

48. National Public Radio, "Morning Edition," April 16, 1996.

49. Ibid., February 2, 1998, and February 25, 2002. There is a women's singles luge event.

50. Leigh, "Evolution," 84.

6. BICYCLING AND THE BLOOMER

1. Most histories of costume mention dress reform to some extent, and several master's theses and Ph.D. dissertations have included the subject. It is a topic much beloved by academic costume historians who respond to counterarguments to the fashion principle. Several nineteenth-century authors wrote on dress reform, and a few books have been written on the subject since. See Stella Mary Newton, *Health, Art, and Reason: Dress Reformers of the Nineteenth Century* (London: John Murray, 1974); Gayle V. Fischer, *Pantaloons and Power: A Nineteenth-Century Dress Reform in the United States* (Kent, Ohio: Kent State University Press, 2001); Patricia A. Cunningham, *Reforming Women's Fashion, 1850–1920* (Kent, Ohio: Kent State University Press, 2003).

2. Fischer, *Pantaloons*, chap. 4, 79–110. Fischer joins others in claiming that the "freedom dress" was based on Turkish dress for women.

3. My thanks to Charlotte Jirousek for her confirmation of this. This outfit was based entirely on Turkish dress, according to Jirousek, rather than just the trousers that most scholars credit as being "Turkish."

4. Quoted in *The Pimlico Companion to Fashion* (London: Pimlico, 1998), 15.

5. Fischer, *Pantaloons*, 50.

6. "Symposium on Women's Dress," *The Arena* 6 (1892), and "The Rational Dress Movement, A Symposium," ibid., 9 (1893).

7. Ibid., 9 (1893): 326.

8. Ibid., 6 (1892): 630.

9. Abba Goold Woolson, *Dress-Reform* (1874; reprint, New York: Arno Press, 1974), ix–x. It is interesting that, over and over again, even the most ardent advocates of any kind of trouser outfits for women labeled them unattractive, even ugly. The mind, it would seem, sees only what it knows and is accustomed to.

10. *The Arena* 9 (1893): 335.

11. Ibid., 336. One is struck by the universality of this observation.

12. Ibid., 9 (1892): 493.

13. Ibid., 502. Here, then, is one of the first statements in the history of trousers for women that actually claims the outfit is attractive rather than ugly.

14. Ibid., 503. The move to reform women's dress was not just an idea of the eastern seaboard. At least two leaders at the symposium came from the Midwest. Frances E. Russell from St. Paul, Minnesota, was named chairman of the Dress Reform Committee of the National Council of Women of the United States; Frances M. Steele came from Chicago.

15. Ibid., 642–43.

16. Ibid., 640.

17. The World's Columbian Exposition of 1893, held a year after the four hundredth anniversary of Columbus's discovery of America, was a huge success. It catapulted the world into the twentieth century, offering products and technology that we still take for granted today: U.S. Postal Service picture postcards, Aunt Jemima pancake syrup, the first commemorative coins, Cream of Wheat and Shredded Wheat, Pabst

beer (it won a blue ribbon), Juicy Fruit gum, carbonated soda, hamburgers, separate amusement areas called midways, Ferris wheels, electricity as universal lighting. It introduced the White City, on which L. Frank Baum patterned his Emerald City of Oz, and it even contracted with a woman architect, Sophia B. Hayden, to design the Women's Building. Frederick Law Olmsted's firm were the consulting landscape architects, and Augustus Saint-Gaudens was the consultant for sculptural design. Among the many websites on the Columbian Exposition, see www.xroads.virginia.edu/~MA96/WCE/legacy.html and www.chicagohs.org/history/expo.html.

18. *Delineator*, May 1889, 311; July 1889, 9.

19. Ibid., May 1890, 341, 355, 358.

20. Ibid., 361, 363.

21. *The Delineator* (November 1894): v.

22. *The Arena* 9 (1893): 306.

23. Ibid., 307.

24. Ibid., 314.

25. Ibid.

26. Stephen Hardy, *How Boston Played* (Boston: Northeastern University Press, 1982), 161, quoting articles from 1892 and 1896.

27. *Harper's Bazar*, June 1, 1895, 443.

28. Ibid., September 7, 1895, 000; May 2, 1896, 387.

29. Ibid., January 18, 1896, 51.

30. Ibid., August 1, 1896, 647.

31. Ibid., August 22, 1896, 707.

32. Ibid., October 24, 1896, 887.

33. Ibid., December 12, 1896, 1039.

34. Ibid., October 12, 1895, 826–27.

35. Ibid.

36. Robert A. Smith, *A Social History of the Bicycle* (New York: American Heritage Press, 1972), gives a good general history; and Sally Sims, "The Bicycle, the Bloomer, and Dress Reform in the 1890s," in Patricia A. Cunningham and Susan Voso Lab, eds., *Dress and Popular Culture* (Bowling Green, Ohio: Popular Press, 1991), 125–43, gives a true view of the use of the bloomer for cycling.

37. Dunlop, a Scot living in Ireland, was not the first to invent the pneumatic tire. An earlier (1846) patent had been taken out, but nothing had been done with the idea. Dunlop, wanting a smoother tricycle ride for his little boy, created the new tire. "Accessory" patents were taken out in 1890, and the Dunlop Tire Company was founded in Dublin. See *Encyclopedia Britannica*, s.v. "Dunlop."

38. Smith, *Social History*, citing *Outing* magazine (June 1892), which predicted that the pneumatic tires would "shove everything to the wall" (20).

39. *Harper's Bazar*, April 25 and May 16, 1896. The advertised price of $85 would amount to $1,736.48 in 2001 dollars; $15 would equal $306.44. The tire ad is for Palmer Tires.

40. *The Delineator* (May 1895): ix. The equivalent costs today would be: $1,965.28 reduced to 1,228.30; $1,670.49 to 884.38; $1,277.43 to 736.98; and $393.06 to 196.53.

41. Ibid. (May 1895): x.

42. *Harper's Bazar*, July 27, 1895. I have deliberately avoided horseback riding in this book because equestrian dress has a history of its own. From at least the sixteenth century on, it was based on men's dress, always exquisitely tailored by men and worn by the affluent only. Riding habits were elegant, fitted, and tailored. Because of their dedicated use, they were free from the embellishments of fashion, and maintained as great a non-fashionable look as was possible in women's wear. Even so, riding habits are readily identifiable as clothing of their own period. The skirt, cut to fit over the knee hooked onto a sidesaddle and droop to cover the other foot as it nestled in the stirrup, was deliberately built lopsided, and designed to create a handsome look while the rider was seated on the horse. When she dismounted and stood, the uneven skirt had to be draped over one arm to prevent it from dragging on the ground. Under this, the rider often wore a pair of equestrian trousers, but these were consistently covered by the skirt. Habits were the clothing of the rich, and remained so. Breeches for women came into use only in the years immediately prior to World War I, and came into fashion for riders in the 1920s. But because the habit was not influenced by the passing fads of sports as they came and went, it does not have a place in this book.

43. Ibid.

44. The term "New Woman" was applied to the privileged few who were being educated in the new colleges and universities, to the even smaller number of professionals who were entering that male-dominated sphere, and to the young women who were employed in the workforce as saleswomen, typists, or teachers. The term often was applied in conjunction with the women's rights workers as well. *Harper's Bazar* reported in 1895 that "a number of the best known advocates of women's rights, including Miss Susan B. Anthony, Mrs. Elizabeth Cady Stanton, Miss Frances Willard. . . and several others, have had their features epitomized in a composite photograph, which, it is claimed, should bear as a title 'The New Woman.'" *Harper's Bazar*, November 23, 1895. These New Women needed new kinds of clothes—simpler, easier to wear and care for; daytime outfits that would take them, in the words of today's advertising, from work into evening.

45. Sims, "The Bicycle," 126.

46. Ibid., 130–31. It is interesting to note that the waves of complaints about back problems only began in the twentieth century, after corsets had finally been abandoned.

47. *Harper's Bazar*, May 2, 1896.

48. Kirk Munroe, "About Bicycles," in Norman W. Bingham Jr., ed., *The Book of Athletics and Out-of-Door Sports* (Boston: Lothrop Publishing Company, 1895), 96–106.

49. *Harper's Bazar*, May 2, 1896.

50. Sally Sims's essay "The Bicycle, the Bloomer, and Dress Reform in the 1890s" (see n. 36) outlines well the position of the bloomer costume as a bicycling choice.

51. *Harper's Bazar*, September 18, 1897, 786–87.

52. Rainy day skirts became popular in the mid-1890s and remained so into the new century. Worn by the athletic woman, often a college girl, they were originally

somewhat daring, but finally made so much sense in an era when skirts trailed on the ground, dragging dirt and refuse along with them, that they were adopted by large numbers of women for walking, and for wet weather in general. It was an obvious choice to use them for bicycling as well.

53. The Eton jacket was cropped to the waist; the Norfolk was an adaptation of menswear, country-bred, tweedy, and replete with pockets, strapping, and a belt; and the basque was a severely form-fitting buttoned bodice that covered the hips.

54. *The Delineator* (November 1895): ii–iv.

55. *Harper's Bazar*, April 25, 1896.

56. Ibid., October 12, 1895, 826.

57. Ibid., July 27, 1895, 595.

58. Ibid. The price of the gloves was the only price given. But when we figure the cost in today's dollars—some $24.50—we begin to realize that the outfits were not for the everyday bicycle rider.

59. All quotations are from "New York Fashions," *Harper's Bazar*, June 13, 1896, 503. Dressmakers at this time were indeed "cheap." Whereas a woman might spend the equivalent of $100 or more for the material for a summer dress, her dressmaker's bill would amount to little more than $10 to $15. Many women earned their living as dressmakers, but almost no one seemed to make a lot doing it. See Patricia Campbell Warner, "It Looks Very Nice Indeed," *Dress 2001* (2002): 23–29.

60. The hat would cost over $50 in today's money. (Perhaps Papa would not scorn it after all.) Her gaiters would cost over $30.50. All quotations from letters of Louise N. Pierce, October 25, 1896, Wellesley College Archives, Wellesley, Mass.

61. Her comments about the roads at Wellesley are not insignificant. It was bicycling that brought about improvements in the condition of roads throughout the entire country, in fact preparing them for the automobile, which was to follow hard on the heels of the bicycle.

62. See Warner, "It Looks Very Nice Indeed."

63. Most of the information in this section comes from nineteenth-century magazines collected in the Bibliothèque Nationale and from the Musée des Arts Decoratifs, both in Paris.

64. *The Arena* (1893): 315.

65. *La Bicyclette*, January 5, 1894.

66. Ibid., 2399. "Elle exhibe sa toilette, / Simple en ses contours coquets. / Et, fiévreusement sportive, / Ses patins à son guidon, / Poursuit sa course hâtive / Sans peur du qu'en dira-t-on."

67. Ibid., 2419. The report is datelined "from London," January 2, 1894.

68. Ibid., January 12, 1894, 2472.

69. *Vélocipède* was the French name for the early bicycle.

70. Ibid., February 2, 1894, 2591; February 23, 1894, 2677.

71. Ibid., March 23, 1894, 2817–18; March 30, 1894, 000–00; April 6, 1894, 2889–90.

72. The Library of the Musée des Arts Décoratifs has a small collection of illustrations of women bicyclists from the 1890s. Four are drawings, the other seven are photographs. They are not offically dated, but seem to range from about 1893 or 1894 to about 1895 or 1896. Three only are bloomer outfits (one has bloomers and a shirtwaist), while at least three others with skirts may have knickers underneath. The skirts seem to be shorter than American ones, hitting just below the knee.

73. Anne Buck, "Foundations of the Active Woman," *La Belle Epoque*, proceedings of the Costume Society Spring Conference (1967): 64.

74. Quoted in Nancy Bradfield, "Cycling in the 1890s," *Costume*, no. 6 (1972): 47.

75. "The Outdoor Woman," *Harper's Bazar*, May 2, 1896.

76. Ibid., February 6, 1897, 111.

77. Mary Sargent Hopkins, "Out of Doors," *The Ladies' World* (February 1898): 10. Courtesy of the Smith College Archives, Northampton, Mass.

PART TWO INTRODUCTION

1. It is perhaps worthwhile to ponder in what way the social commentators a century hence will regard the zeitgeist of our own time. We have a tendency to recoil from the limitations placed on women a century or more ago, and we certainly remain bemused by the clothing they wore. Women today feel that we have achieved an advanced status, and we are proud of our achievements. But a century from now, women will almost assuredly be equally aghast that we were so smug at the turn of the twenty-first century. After all, they may say, we had been striving for equality for 150 years and still were able to earn only seventy-five cents to every man's dollar. And the clothes! Young women's were tight, sleazy, revealing cleavages both front and back, at a time when young men's clothes were looser and more covering than perhaps they ever had been before. This is freedom from men's domination, they might ask? This is equality?

2. Ellen W. Gerber, *The American Woman in Sport* (Reading, Mass.: Addison-Wesley, 1974), 4–5, 12.

3. Lizzie Southgate Parker, handwritten document, Smith College Archives.

4. Gerber, *American Woman*, 12.

5. However ludicrous this may seem at a time when young women routinely wear to class and everywhere else strapless stretch tops that bare their bellies this same rule persisted well into the mid-twentieth century. Women had to wear raincoats (even in the bright sunshine) to cover up their gym suits well into the 1970s and 1980s.

6. Gertrude Walker, "Report," Smith College Archives.

7. Lizzie Southgate Parker, "Physical Culture at Smith," Smith College Archives.

8. It is interesting to note that Smith College has been a successful fund-raiser from its early years. At the time the gymnasium funds were being raised, the college was only thirteen years old, and its total alumnae body can't have numbered many more than 1,300, figured on the basis of one hundred students per class—probably a generous estimate for the time.

9. "History of the Physical Education Department," Mount Holyoke College Archives.

10. Parker, "Physical Culture."

11. Oberlin College claims the first woman graduate, in 1841. The curriculum for women at Oberlin, however, was significantly different from the men's. Essentially, women were educated to be the helpmeets of the young men who trained there for the missionary field. Women were taught housewifery skills and genteel accomplishments, not so very different from the curriculum of the ladies' seminaries of the period. Women were tolerated (barely) in the early years of many of the great land grant universities, and though they were accepted into many of the classes offered, they had to be dedicated and determined if they were to get an education. The prejudice died hard, lasting well into the final decades of the twentieth century in fields such as medicine, architecture, and law. Only since the early 1990s have women outnumbered men in universities and colleges, some 54 to 46 percent by the beginning of the twenty-first century. Overall, even by the first decades of the twentieth century, only a tiny percentage of men and women went to colleges and universities. In 1870, when the total population of the United States was 38,155,505, 11,000 women were enrolled in U.S. colleges; men outnumbered them 4 or 5 to 1. Few women actually graduated; male graduates outnumbered women 7 to 1. By 1900, out of a total population of 74,607,225, 85,000 women were enrolled; by 1920, 283,000. Anne J. MacLachlan, *The Inclusion of Women in American Higher Education: Institutional Adaptation and Resistance*, population statistics, Inter-university Consortium for Political and Social Research (ICPSR), http://fisher.lib.virginia.edu/census.

7. TROUSER WEARING

1. The name "slops" had been given to very baggy knee-covering breeches at the beginning of the seventeenth century. The later sailors' slops retained the fullness created by gathers at the waist but were straight-cut in the leg and fell above the ankle.

2. The troupes of masked players with their set cast of characters and their witty, skillfully improvised dialogue dated back to the sixteenth century. The name commedia dell'arte came about in the eighteenth century. A series of illustrations (at McGill University) made from bird feathers by Dionisio Managgio in 1618 shows one figure, Trapolino, in an outfit that looks as if it dated from the twentieth century, with his short jacket with standard coat sleeves and full-length trousers. Other characters in the series also wear simple, gently fitted trousered suits. Another series by the Englishman John Collins, active in the early 1680s, depicts "Signor Scaramouche and His Company," with Scaramouche himself wearing another of these simple trousered suits. Others wear trousers as well, but as part of much more decorated or stylized costumes. By the eighteenth century, Claude Gillot, François Joullain, and others also depicted the comic characters in several series of engravings. Perhaps the most lasting images were the Meissen figurines of the commedia, which were copied and produced by many other companies from the early eighteenth century right up to the present. See Eleonora Luciano, *The Mask of Comedy: The Art of Italian Commedia* (Louisville: J. B. Speed Art Museum, 1990).

3. Diana De Marly, *Fashion for Men* (London: B. T. Batsford, 1985), 72.

4. Quoted in Elizabeth Ewing, *History of Children's Costume* (New York: Charles Scribner's Sons, 1977), 46–47. Also see Clare Rose, *Children's Clothes* (London: B. T. Batsford, 1989), 48–50.

5. See Ewing, *History*, 48–51; and De Marly, *Fashion for Men*, 72.

6. Rose, *Children's Clothes* 48–50. Rose's reference to Locke (who died in 1704) cites a 1787 German fashion magazine. Rose claims that the skeleton suit "was firmly associated with English tastes and the English way of life." Even François Boucher, French to the core, admits that "under the influence of the English," the dress of eighteenth-century children ceased to be that of miniature adults. François Boucher, *Histoire du Costume* (Paris: Flammarion, 1983), 304.

7. Rose, *Children's Clothes*, 50.

8. The growing demand for and importance of cotton in the eighteenth century cannot be ignored in any history of the period. These cotton baby dresses, affordable only to the rich (most children of the time continued to wear the same clothing as their parents; for little girls that meant chemises, stays, and petticoats), marked the beginning of the demand for cotton clothing. The Industrial Revolution began as a result of the demand for textiles: all the inventions that initiated it were textile industry machines. The cotton gin enabled cotton to be processed more cheaply in the West, led to the establishment of cotton plantations in the United States, and eventually to the sharp increase in the slave trade, which led to the Civil War almost one hundred years after the first machines were invented to aid the mass production of cotton.

9. Zoffany's *Lord Willoughby and His Family* (ca. 1775) is an example. There are three children in this portrait of the family gathered around a tea table. All wear the same white dress. One little boy is sneaking a cookie, the other is running through the room pulling a toy horse on wheels, and the docile little girl perches beside her mother.

10. Scholars generally agree about this. Alison Carter writes, "There is scant evidence for female drawers being widely worn in Europe before the nineteenth century." Alison Carter, *Underwear: The Fashion History* (New York: Drama Books, 1992), 14. Boucher informs us that drawers had been obligatory in the theater since 1760 but had been lost to general usage by the end of the century; *Histoire*, 304.

11. C. Willett Cunnington and Phillis Cunnington, *The History of Underclothes* (1951; reprint, New York: Dover, 1992), 110.

12. Ewing, *History*, 65.

13. Pierre Dufay, *Le Pantalon feminin*, quoted in Anne Wood Murray, "The Bloomer Costume and Exercise Suits," in *Waffen- und Kostümekunde* (Munich: Deutscher Kunstverlag, 1982), 113.

14. Cunnington and Cunnington, *Underclothes*, 110, quoting from the *Glenbervie Journals* (1811).

15. See Charlotte Jirousek, "More than Oriental Splendor: European and Ottoman Headgear, 1380–1580," *Dress* 22 (1995): 22–33, for an overview of the Ottoman Empire's early influence on European dress.

16. The story of the British East India Company is one of commercial and militaristic aggression and expansion. By the mid-eighteenth century, England had taken over the governance of India and was reaping the benefits. Perceptions of that history are shaped by Hollywood versions of Indian history, usually romanticizing if not glorifying the dauntless Victorians. Certainly Queen Victoria relished her title, empress of India. It came to her courtesy of the trade expansion efforts established by her ancestor Queen Elizabeth I in 1600.

17. Palempores were large printed and painted cotton hangings or bed coverings made in India, intricate versions of what later came to be known as chintz. First imported into Europe in the seventeenth century, by the eighteenth century the most popular ones had Tree of Life designs surrounded by patterned borders.

18. See Jirousek, "More than Oriental Splendor."

19. See Aileen Ribeiro, *The Art of Dress* (New Haven: Yale University Press, 1995), 222–28, for a discussion of Oriental influences, especially Turkish, on clothing in paintings.

20. Ibid., 222.

21. Banyans were loose coats meant to be worn at home. Often they were made of luxurious fabrics—silk, velvet, brocades—lined with fur to ward off the drafts of lofty rooms. Many men had their portraits painted in these, too. A famous American example is John Singleton Copley's portrait of Nicholas Boyston in the Museum of Fine Arts in Boston. Banyans evolved into dressing gowns in the nineteenth century.

22. Jane Ashelford, *The Art of Dress* (New York: Harry N. Abrams, 1996), 102.

8. THE RISE OF INTEREST IN EXERCISE FOR WOMEN

1. Geoffrey Squire, *Dress and Society, 1560–1970* (New York: Viking Press, 1974), 159.

2. See Nancy Woloch, *Women and the American Experience* (New York: Alfred A. Knopf, 1984), chaps. 5 and 6, "Sarah Hale and the Ladies Magazine" and "Promoting the Women's Sphere, 1800–1860."

3. Lois W. Banner, *American Beauty* (Chicago: University of Chicago Press, 1983), 62.

4. Rachel H. Kemper, *Costume* (New York: Newsweek Books, 1977), 125.

5. Squire, *Dress*, 159. "The expansive sleeve" is a reference to the huge, exuberant balloon sleeves of the late 1820s and 1830s, which grew to an expanse not matched until the mid-1890s, then collapsed to nothing, as if pricked by a pin.

6. Sarah J. Hale, "How To Begin," *Godey's* (July 1841): 41.

7. Quoted in Stephanie L. Twin, "Jock and Jill: Aspects of Women's Sport History in America, 1870–1940" (Ph.D. diss., Rutgers University, 1978), 87, 88.

8. Anne Wood Murray, "The Bloomer Costume and Exercise Suits," in *Waffen- und Kostümkunde* (Munich: Deutscher Kunstverlag, 1982), 115.

9. Catharine Beecher, "1863 Oration at Seminary Anniversary," Mount Holyoke College Archives and Special Collections.

10. See Barbara Welter, "The Feminization of American Religion: 1800–1860," in Mary Hartman and Lois W. Banner, eds., *Clio's Consciousness Raised* (New York: Harper and Row, 1974), 137–57.

11. Woloch, *Women and the American Experience*, 122.

12. Ibid., 129.

13. Katherine Kish Sklar, *Catharine Beecher: A Study in American Domesticity* (New York: W. W. Norton and Co., 1973), 151–54. The material on Beecher is from this source unless otherwise noted.

14. The role of home economics changed during the last quarter of the twentieth century, taking it out of the Beecher mode in an attempt to bring it into a more modern

world that was seeking equality in expectation for women rather than the separate but equal realm it had occupied before. Perhaps its very success in educating women was the cause of its decline: finally, women really were being educated equally to men in all fields, so colleges and universities could no longer justify an educational area dedicated to domesticity. Today, many home economics departments and institutions are closing or being folded into more generic fields: sociology, psychology, social work, food science, architecture, and the like.

15. Ibid., 160.

16. Catharine Beecher, "On the Peculiar Responsibilities of American Women," reprinted in Nancy F. Cott, ed., *Root of Bitterness* (New York: E. P. Dutton, 1972), 174, 177.

17. Sklar, *Catharine Beecher*, 206.

18. Fred Eugene Leonard, *History of Physical Education* (Philadelphia: Lea and Febiger, 1923), 231.

19. The image in *Godey's* ([August 1848]: 112) copied, virtually line for line, the earlier image from *The Young Girl's Book*. In the days before copyright laws, this was a customary practice.

20. See Murray, "Bloomer Costume," 114.

21. Woloch, *Women and the American Experience*, 127.

22. See Helen Lefkowitz Horowitz, *Alma Mater* (Amherst: University of Massachusetts, Press, 1993), chap. 1, "Plain Though Very Neat: Mount Holyoke," for a discussion of early schools for women, including Troy Seminary, and the history of Mount Holyoke.

23. Woloch, *Women and the American Experience*, 127.

24. *Holyoke Daily Transcript and Telegram*, Mount Holyoke centennial year supplement, May 8, 1937, quoting a letter written by Mary Lyon. Mount Holyoke College Archives and Special Collections.

25. Mount Holyoke College Archives and Special Collections. See Patricia Campbell Warner, "Washed again today, the skin was gone from my hands': Doing the Laundry in Women's Colleges, 1840–1890," *Dress* 30 (2003): 38–47.

26. Mount Holyoke College Archives and Special Collections.

27. Letters of Lucy T. Goodale, ibid.

28. No date, no publishers, but used until about 1867 at the seminary. Ibid.

29. "Teachers' Book of Duties," no date, ibid.

30. See www.oberlin.edu/~EOG/LucyStonewalkathonTour/Delphine%20Hanna.

31. Unless otherwise noted, information on Dio Lewis is from Leonard, *History of Physical Education*, 255–62.

32. Quoted ibid., 258–59. The article was written by Thomas Wentworth Higginson.

33. Ibid., 258–59.

34. Dio Lewis. *The New Gymnastics for Men, Women, and Children*, 10th ed. (Boston: Fields and Osgood, & Co., 1869), 18.

35. The high-cut sleeve seam was unusual in the 1860s. Characteristically at this time, sleeve seams fell off the shoulder in a continuation of the bodice line. Lewis stip-

ulated the higher seam to allow for freer movement of the arm, which would have been hampered by the fashionable cut.

36. Undated letter, Mount Holyoke College Archives and Special Collections.

37. Linda Martin, *The Way We Wore* (New York: Charles Scribner's Sons, 1978), 15.

38. *Godey's* (January 1864): 105.

8. INNOVATION AT WELLESLEY

1. *The Delineator Autumn Catalogue* (1889): 16.

2. All quotations are from *Notes on Mr. Durant's Sermon on "The Spirit of the College"* (Boston: Frank Wood, Printer, 1890), probably delivered on September 23, 1877.

3. The first year, 315 students were enrolled; by 1881, there were 450. Wellesley College Calendars, 1876–77, 1881–82. For more about Henry Fowle Durant and Wellesley history, see Helen Lefkowitz Horowitz, *Alma Mater* (Amherst: University of Massachusetts Press, 1984).

4. Florence Converse, *The Story of Wellesley* (Boston: Little, Brown, 1915), 37.

5. Linda K. Vaughan, "A Century of Rowing at Wellesley," a paper presented at the Annual Conference of the North American Society for Sports History, April 18, 1975.

6. Archival photographs at Wellesley College show either six-plus-one, seven-plus-one, or eight-plus-one configurations, all dating from 1879 to the early 1880s. The "one" girl faced the rowers in the cox position; I assume she acted as coxswain.

7. Jean Glasscock, ed., *Wellesley College, 1875–1975: A Century of Women* (Wellesley, Mass.: Wellesley College, 1975), 242.

8. Vaughan, "Century of Rowing"; Converse, *Story of Wellesley*, 216.

9. Issues of *The Delineator* from the early 1880s show several "blouse costumes" for children, including a sailor dress ([June 1884]: 438–39), but none for adults. Basques of various lengths were the common style. This continued at least as late as March 1894 (xxxviii), but by this time similar two-piece outfits, usually with sailor collars, were appearing for "misses" up to age sixteen.

10. Lucy Hunt, *The Handbook of Light Gymnastics* (Boston: Lee and Shepard Publishers, 1885), 80–87.

11. The Wellesley "Specials" were non-degree students, usually older, often teachers, who returned to school for further education. Some were mothers, others were single—this a century before the phenomenon of returning, older, mostly female students which we now think of as a recent innovation.

12. All the coeducational institutions I visited which offered early team sports for men had photographic evidence of these athletic jerseys. They were popular and widely used in all sports settings, not just academic ones.

13. *Wellesley (Mass.) Courant* (college edition), June 21, 1889.

14. All quotations in this section are from the *Wellesley Courant*, June 21, 1889.

15. Chauncey Depew was a famous orator of his day. His fame followed him well into the middle of the twentieth century by way of a childhood nonsense ditty, one line of which ran "Chauncey Pew will speak to you at two o'clock tonight."

16. *Boston Daily Globe*, June 8, 1894.

17. "In the Realm of Sport and Athletics," *Ladies' Every Saturday*, August 24, 1895, 12.

18. It is interesting to note that although all three of these other colleges also had lakes on campus, none had an official rowing program. Interesting, too, is the fact that competition was frowned on in every realm but clothing.

19. All the colleges for women reiterated these tenets. Many references are found in the archives at each school. See Patricia Campbell Warner, "Public and Private: Clothing the American Women for Sport and Physical Education, 1860–1940," Ph.D. diss., University of Minnesota, 1986, 79–80. A clipping in the Wellesley Archives further upholds this claim. Dated 1893 (source unknown) and written by Grace Weld Soper, "Wellesley Float '93" mentions the crews floating across the lake "without any attempt at racing." Soper also suggested that "to a thoughtful observer it was . . . an effort to improve the health of the college students by systematic out-door exercise. The perfect time of the oars, the erect carriage of the rowers, and their ease of motion showed both gymnastic training and careful coaching. All the muscles of the body were called into play, and especially in the boats with the sliding seats the exercise produced the greatest harmony of motion."

20. *Boston Daily Globe*, June 8, 1894.

21. Vaughan, "A Century of Rowing at Wellesley," quoting Helen Shafer in "The President's Report," Wellesley College, 1893.

22. *Boston Daily Globe*, June 8, 1894.

23. *Legenda, the Wellesley Magazine* (June 1893): 457.

24. *Boston Herald*, June 12, 1895.

25. Ibid., June 17, 1897.

26. Mount Holyoke College Archives and Special Collections, photo collection.

27. On consideration, it is not surprising that the impetus for the suits came from the students themselves. As is still true today, young women of college age were the group most devoted to the passing vagaries of fashion and most concerned with "new" clothing.

10. THE DEBUT OF THE GYM SUIT

1. It didn't occur to me as a high school student to wonder about this inequity, or to wonder where the teachers' outfit had come from and why it was so different, hygienic aspects aside, from ours. Now, of course, I understand that it was the regulation physical education uniform that many teachers who had graduated from established university programs wore. My two high school phys ed teachers, Miss Martinson and Miss Redfern, both wore navy tunics over their white blouses, but the younger, prettier one who "left to get married" had a rosy red one that we all loved to see her wear.

2. Mabel Lee, *Memories of a Bloomer Girl (1894–1924)* (Washington, D.C.: American Alliance for Health, Physical Education, and Recreation, 1977), 19. The dates Lee gives indicate that exercise was a component of the curriculum from the opening year of each college.

3. It is noteworthy, almost astonishing, that many schools, from Rockford College in Illinois, to Wellesley, to girls' schools in Missouri and Nebraska, to Mills College in

California and even Oberlin College in Ohio (older than Mount Holyoke, but with a women's division that was established later and patterned on the Mount Holyoke model), all have Mount Holyoke somewhere in their pedigree. The students trained as teachers at Mount Holyoke scattered to the new schools, and they took Mary Lyon's precepts with them to establish strong new educational systems for young women across the country. Another reason for concentrating on these schools is that they all have remarkable archives.

4. I chose the University of Toronto for a number of reasons. First, it is my own alma mater. Second, its history reflects what was going on elsewhere, in schools such as the University of Michigan and the University of Minnesota. And as a Canadian school, it provides some broader North American balance.

5. *Torontonensis* (1900), 69.

6. Historically, the University of Toronto is an amalgamation of several liberal arts colleges, a number of them historically church-based: Trinity (Anglican); St. Michael's (Roman Catholic); and Victoria (originally Methodist, now United Church of Canada). Each college retains its separate identity, not just for students' living arrangements but for academic subjects as well, much as in the great English universities.

7. *Torontonensis* (1903), 248.

8. Persis Harlow McCurdy, "The History of Physical Training at Mount Holyoke College," *American Physical Education Review*, 14, no. 3 (March 1909): 146. Zouave trousers were patterned after the pants of the North African Zouave regiment in the French army, which fought so valiantly and fearlessly in the mid-century Algerian war and later. The trousers were baggy and full, falling to mid-calf, and worn with short bolero jackets; both were adapted from North African native dress, and were usually navy and red in combination. In the American Civil War, Zouave troops were formed in New York and other states in homage to the courage of the French Zouaves; these American men also wore the colorful Zouave uniform. Although the soldiers of the time adopted the unusual outfit, it was never brought into civilian wear for men. For women, it was another story. They snatched up that bolero jacket, making it the hit of the 1850s and 1860s. It became known in women's fashions as simply "the zouave." Even the trousers were adopted by women, but, not surprisingly in light of what we know of the period, they found their place more or less hidden away in the new gymnasiums of the time. Eventually, that loose, baggy, crotch-at-the-knees cut became the standard bloomer bottom of the basketball gym suit of the 1890s.

9. Mount Holyoke College Archives and Special Collections.

10. For more about Cornelia Clapp and her influence at Mount Holyoke, see Patricia Campbell Warner and Margaret S. Ewing, "Wading in the Water: Women Aquatic Biologists Coping with Clothing, 1877–1945," *BioScience* 52, no. 1 (January 2002): 97–104. That article is modified here in chapter 11.

11. Cornelia M. Clapp, *Manual of Gymnastics* (1883), 33. Mount Holyoke College Archives.

12. This leaves open the question, did the Wellesley crew outfits have drawers too?

13. Harriet Isabel Ballintine, *The History of Physical Training at Vassar College* (Poughkeepsie, N.Y.: Lansing & Broas, Printers, 1915), 6–7, Vassar College Archives.

14. Florence Woolsey Hazzard, "Heart of Oak: The Story of Eliza Moser," insert 6, 5, Bentley Historical Library, University of Michigan.

15. Mr. McGee's Scrap Books, "Muscular Maids," no newspaper, no date (late 1880s), University of California–Berkeley University Archives. This little tale continues with a converation between two of the gymnasts: "'Yes, if one could only be as free as this all the time.' 'Well,' the other answers, 'and why can't we, you and I?' They look at each other, the horror of a short-skirted promenade down Broadway making mischief in their eyes. . . . And still the question is unanswered, why." It is obvious that the daring new unskirted gymnastic dress was unthinkable outside the gymnasium itself.

16. Ibid., no date (1888).

17. *The Arena* 7 (1893): 76.

18. All information in this chapter not otherwise cited is from the archives of selected private and public colleges and universities throughout the United States, including bulletins, calendars, published and unpublished histories, letters, photographs, scrapbooks, yearbooks, and the garments themselves. The schools include Mount Holyoke College, Rockford College, Smith College, Wellesley College, Vassar College, the University of California–Berkeley and Los Angeles, Iowa State University, the University of Michigan, the University of Minnesota, the University of North Carolina at Greensboro, Stanford University, and the University of Wisconsin.

19. The University of Michigan is a good example. Women's physical education officially began there in 1905, but a basketball club was organized by women students as early as 1893, the year after the game was introduced. *The University of Michigan: An Encyclopedic Survey*, vol. 4, pt. 9 (Ann Arbor: University of Michigan Press, 1958), 1994–2004.

20. See Patricia Campbell Warner, "Public and Private: Men's Influence on American Women's Dress for Sport and Physical Education," *Dress* 24 (1988): 48–55, for a further discussion of this point.

21. Orrin Leslie Elliott, *Stanford University: The First Twenty-five Years* (Stanford: Stanford University Press, 1937), 197–98.

22. Ibid.

23. Warner, "Public and Private," 51.

24. A number of schools mention her visit in their archives, but reports vary as to which she visited first. It is certain that she gave demonstrations at Wellesley, and gave instruction at Vassar, Smith, Mount Holyoke, Bryn Mawr, and Radcliffe. Ballintine, *History of Physical Training*, 15, 18.

25. *Boston Sunday Herald* magazine, February 10, 1907, 7, Sophia Smith Collection, Smith College.

26. Almost invariably the color was navy or black. One exception: the Valentine Museum in Richmond, Virginia, has a maroon serge two-piece gymnasium suit, ca. 1905–1910 in its collection (v.72.351.5.a,b). My thanks to Colleen Callahan for this information.

27. Second Annual Catalogue of the State Normal and Industrial School, Greensboro, N.C., 1893–94, 33. The actual cost that year was listed as $5.75; by 1895–96, the

catalogue claimed the total to be "not more than $5.00." In 2002 dollars this would amount to approximately $100.

28. There is little research to date into the companies that manufactured and supplied gym suits to the schools, though what there is so far bears this supposition out. Wright & Ditson and Spalding are two of the companies that manufactured garments for physical education in the 1920s through the 1940s; the earliest extant garments have no labels, or if any, that of a store, such as Stearn's in Boston.

29. *Detroit Free Press,* November 2, 1896.

30. Department of Special Collections, Stanford University Libraries, photographs 1208, 1209, and 1219.

31. *Third Annual Catalogue* (1894–95), State Normal and Industrial School, Greensboro, N.C., 36. This outfit in its entirety cost no more than five dollars.

32. Leonhard Felix Fuld, "Gymnastic Costume for Women," *American Physical Education Review* 15 (November 1910): 574.

33. Leonard Felix Fuld, "Gymnastic Costume for Women. II," *American Physical Education Review* 16 (November 1911): 522–23.

34. Fuld, "Gymnastic Costume," 574.

35. Ibid., 573, 578.

36. Ibid., 574. By 1910, many high schools throughout the country had physical education programs. Of these, many required only loose street clothing, since there were few facilities for changing in any of the schools, although some with gymnasiums did demand appropriate gymnasium dress.

37. Florence Bolton. "Women's Dress in Exercise," *American Physical Education Review* 15 (1910): 338–41.

38. For a history of the English version of gymnastic or sport uniform, see Patricia Campbell Warner, "The Gym Slip: The Origins of the English Schoolgirl Tunic," *Dress* 22 (1996): 45–58.

39. Fuld, "Gymnastic Costume," 576.

40. Fuld, "Gymnastic Costume. II," 521.

41. Fuld, "Gymnastic Costume," 573–75.

42. Ibid., 575–76.

43. Annette Kellerman. "Why and How Girls Should Swim," *Ladies' Home Journal* (August 1910): 11. It took a century after it was devised for male gymnasts for a similar outfit to be generally accepted for women; not until the 1990s did we see women outdoors running in such apparel. As noted earlier, even as recently as 1985, Anne White scandalized Wimbledon by appearing in a white bodysuit. Patricia Campbell Warner, "Public and Private: Clothing the American Woman for Sport and Physical Education, 1860–1940," Ph.D. diss., University of Minnesota, 1986, 124.

44. The wool suits, though in theory washable, were not. Indeed, as we have seen from the Fuld and Bolton articles, and from several references in letters and journals, they lasted through the two years they were needed by the girls at school, uncleaned in any way.

45. Eleanor Edwards to Mildred Howard, November 6, 1947, Mount Holyoke College Archives.

46. Letter to the author from Claire Masters, Waco, Texas, September 18, 1990, and conversations with other Texans. Masters recalled her years at North Hollywood Junior High School in Los Angeles and North Junior High School in Waco. The shorts, she reported, "were cut straight and brief" and "were every bit as brief as those worn today." It is interesting to note the intrusion of domesticity, so characteristic of the period, in the seemingly universal requirement of embroidered names.

47. As recently as the 1960s, when the question of topless bathing suits was first raised, several cities in the United States, including Minneapolis, found to their embarrassment that they were still legally bound by statutes prohibiting bare legs on public beaches. Needless to say, these were laws that had been happily ignored for decades.

48. Mount Holyoke College has a unique collection of women's gymnastic dress dating from the 1860s to the 1980s.

49. Much of this information is anecdotal. Nevertheless, many women from all parts of the country have reported that they had to wear standard gym suits in high school—even those with baggy bloomer bottoms that hit just above the knee—in the 1970s. Most of the holdouts were parochial schools, where, if anywhere, one would expect to find a clinging conservatism.

11. TAKING EXERCISE CLOTHES TO NEW PLACES

1. See Patricia A. Cunningham, *Reforming Women's Fashion, 1850–1920* (Kent, Ohio: Kent State University Press, 2003), for an extended discussion of the dress reform movement.

2. "Dress Reform at the World's Fair," *American Review of Reviews*, April 7, 1893, www.boondocksnet.com/expos/wfe_1893_amrr_dress_reform.html (accessed March 13, 2004).

3. Information on Mrs. Gatty and her clothing comes from R. F. Scagel, formerly a marine biologist at the University of British Columbia. My sincere thanks to James W. Markham of the University of California–Santa Barbara for this connection. Mrs. Gatty's comments were probably originally published in *British sea-weeds. Drawn from Professor Harvey's "Phycologia britannica." With descriptions, an amateur's synopsis, rules for laying out sea-weeds, an order for arranging them in the herbarium, and an appendix of new species. By Mrs. Alfred Gatty* (London: Bell and Daldy, 1872). Scagel quoted Mrs. Gatty's recollections on the verso of the title page of his treatise *Marine Algae of British Columbia and Northern Washington*, Part 1, *Chlorophyceae (Green Algae)* (Ottawa: Queen's Printer, 1966).

4. See Mary Stevens's account in the Mount Holyoke college yearbook, *Llamarada* (1897), 59. Louis Agassiz, the preeminent biologist in nineteenth-century America, was director of the Museum of Comparative Zoology at Harvard.

5. Helen A. Padykula, "Christiana Smith, 1893–1983," memorial in *The Anatomical Record* 210 (1984): 180–83.

6. See June Swann, *Shoes* (London: M. T. Batsford, 1982), 41–42; Colin McDowell, *Shoes: Fashion and Fantasy* (New York: Rizzoli, 1989), 143.

7. Sophia Smith Collection, Smith College.

8. Cornelia Clapp to Ann H. Morgan, July 4, 1924, Mount Holyoke College Archives and Special Collections.

12. THE MERGING OF PUBLIC AND PRIVATE

1. See http://wiwi.essortment.com/americanfootbal_rwff.htm (accessed March 17, 2004).

2. Munsingwear began to manufacture its knitwear at the same time that jersey was becoming popular in England for the same kinds of clothing and even, as we have seen, for tennis dresses for women. See http://www.mnhs.org/library/findaids/00206.html#a2 (accessed March 28, 2004).

3. Materials on Jantzen from the company website, www.jantzenswim.com/hframe.html, and from the Smithsonian Institution website, http://americanhistory.is.edu/archives/d9233.htm. For an in-depth history of the mass production of clothing in the United States, see Claudia B. Kidwell and Margaret C. Christman, *Suiting Everyone: The Democratization of Clothing in America* (Washington, D.C.: Smithsonian Institution Press, 1974).

4. See, by Valerie Steele, *Paris Fashion* (New York: Oxford University Press, 1988), 244–252; and "Chanel in Context," in Juliet Ash and Elizabeth Wilson, eds., *Chic Thrills* (Stanford: University of California Press, 1993), 118–126.

5. See Patricia Campbell Warner, "The Americanization of Fashion: Sportswear, the Movies, and the 1930s," in Linda Welters and Patricia A. Cunningham, eds., *Twentieth-Century Fashion: A Book of Readings* (New York: Berg Publishers, 2005).

6. Movie magazines were introduced in 1910 by Vitagraph Studio. This "innovative kind of fiction publication dedicated to a new audience, motion picture enthusiasts. . . [unleashed] fan interest and activities in ways. . . [the editors] could not have dreamed of—and that they became wary of." Kathryn H. Fuller, *At the Picture Show* (Washington, D.C.: Smithsonian Institution Press, 1996), 133. See also Anthony Slide, "Early Film Magazines: An Overview," in *Aspects of Film History Prior to 1920* (Metuchen, N.J.: Scarecrow Press, 1978). There are many general histories of American film, but a fine compilation may be found in Charles Harpole, general ed., *History of American Cinema* (New York: Charles Scribner's Sons, 1990).

7. See www.silentsmajority.com/PhotoGallery6/bb10.htm for several photos of Mack Sennett "Bathing Beauties" from about 1915 to 1925, including Gloria Swanson and Marie Prevost in 1916. Here, Swanson wears the cotton bathing dress of the time, with bloomers and a skirt, but Prevost wears the newer Olympics-style wool knit suit. "Phlirtatious Phyllis Haver, c. 1915" is also pictured, wearing a cotton Empire-waist bathing dress with narrow straps, bloomers pushed up high and tight, and a wet skirt draped above them to reveal a rounded bare thigh.

8. When the feminist revolution sent women off to work in unprecedented numbers in the 1970s, the question of their wearing trousers arose for debate. During that decade, just about the only women who wore trousers to work were secretaries and other non-professional workers. Indeed, more than one commentator noted that you could tell a woman's status by looking at the clothes she wore to the office. *The Women's*

Dress for Success Book categorically denied that trousers were acceptable for business. The higher the position in a company, the less likely the woman was to wear trousers, even into the early 1990s.

9. Anne Edwards, *A Remarkable Woman* (New York: William Morrow & Co., 1985), 98–99. When Hepburn wore pants on the set of her first movie, *Bill of Divorcement* (1932), George Cukor, her director, complained.

INDEX

INDEX

PATRICIA CAMPBELL WARNER was born and educated in Toronto, Canada, receiving her B.A. in art and archaeology at the University of Toronto. Her M.A. and Ph.D. in design and the history of design were completed at the University of Minnesota almost thirty years later. She has been a historian of dress at the University of Massachusetts Amherst since 1988, currently as professor in the Theater Department. She has published widely in scholarly journals and books on various aspects of the history of dress, including jewelry, slave clothing, and the movies, but her major focus has been the subject of this book, women's clothing for sports. Warner is a Fellow of The Costume Society of America.